Mold Illness and Mold Remediation Made Simple

Removing Mold Toxins From Bodies and Sick Buildings

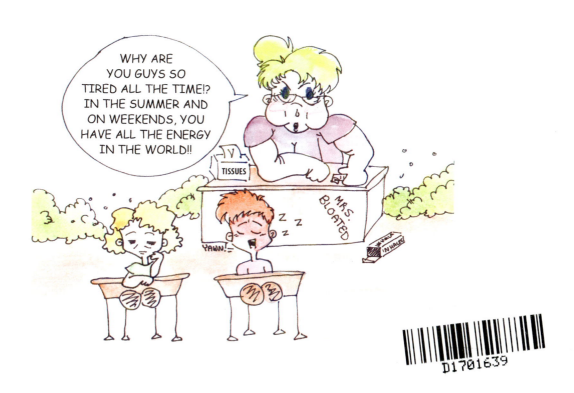

James Schaller, MD, CMR
Gary Rosen, PhD, CIE

Artwork by Jamie Joyce
Book & Cover Design by Philip Chow
Book Production by Ronald Gombach

Hope Academic Press
Tampa, Florida
Copyright © 2005 James Schaller, M.D.
All Rights Reserved
ISBN 0-9773971-2-2

To the millions suffering from mold illness who have been ignored ...

And to Marianne Schaller for listening to the ill.

The medical ideas, health thoughts, building health comments, products and any claims made about specific illnesses, diseases, and causes of health problems in this book, have not been evaluated by the FDA, the USDA, OSHA, CDC, NIH, NIMH or the AMA. Never assume any United States medical body or society, or the majority of American physicians endorse any comment in this book. No comments in this book are approved by any government agency or medical body or society. No comments in this book are meant to diagnose, treat, cure or prevent disease. The information provided in this book is for informational purposes only and is not intended as a substitute for the advice from your physician or other health care professional. This book is not intended to replace or adjust any information contained on or in any product label or packaging. You should not use the information in this book for the diagnosis or treatment of any health problem or as an endorsement of any prescription medication or other treatment. You should consult with a health care professional before deciding on any diagnosis, or initiating any treatment plan of any kind. Please do not start any diet, exercise or supplementation program, or take any type of nutrient, herb, or medication without clear consultation with your licensed health care provider. If you have or suspect you might have a health problem, please do not use this book to replace a prompt consultation with your health care provider(s).

Do You Know

- Mold toxins decrease awareness and insight?
- Mold chemicals can increase cancer, strokes and heart attacks?
- Mold chemicals in the air can increase irritability and cause moodiness?
- Mold can decrease your insight and can make your IQ fall?
- Mold can hurt your ability to relate and get along with people?
- Mold chemicals in the air can make you foggy, tired, bloated and feeling flat?
- You can often spot mold with a little training?
- Mold toxins can hurt virtually every organ in the body?
- How to quickly identify a dangerous mold remediator?
- Most air filters in homes, schools and businesses are junk and ineffective?

For these reasons and many others, you must read this book.

Meet the Authors

A top physician and master builder team up to clearly help you recover from indoor mold exposure. If you can find a smarter and clearer book on mold, buy it!

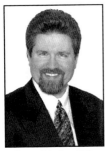
James Schaller, M.D.

Drs. Schaller and Rosen have written or co-authored seven previous books on mold illness treatment and mold-related construction defects, along with dozens of scientific and educational publications. They have written about treating mold illness, removing mold toxins, proof of mold health effects, mold testing, school indoor air quality, disaster restoration, and specialized lab testing, which show how mold toxins can cause obesity, mood problems, fatigue, concentration difficulties, cancer and hormone abnormalities. They are committed to restoring health to bodies and buildings quickly and efficiently.

Dr. Schaller is a prolific writer with over thirty innovative medical treatments. He specializes in patients who lack solutions. His initial training in child and adult psychiatry now includes research and publications in over fifteen areas of medicine. Dr. Schaller is the co-discoverer of a functional cure for a rare blood cancer which is the standard around the world. He is the author of fifteen books, including the recently released, **When You Are Losing Your Mind Over Your Child: 100 Real Solutions!**

Dr. Schaller is also the co-author of the 600-page **Mold Warriors: Fighting America's Hidden Health Threat**, and is one of the few physicians in the United States successfully treating mold toxin illness in children and adults.

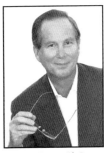
Gary Rosen, Ph.D.

Dr. Rosen is a biochemist with training under a Nobel Prize winning researcher at UCLA. He is the author of **Mold Remediation and Mold Toxins: What You Need to Know Before Hiring a Remediation Contractor**. He is an expert mold remediator of homes, schools and large commercial buildings, and is gifted at finding reasonable and cost effective clean-up solutions. He and his family are vulnerable to indoor toxic mold. He understands its effects first hand.

Together, the authors have certifications in mold testing, mold remediation and indoor environmental evaluation.

Why Comic Illustrations?

Our patients and clients explain they are very busy and also struggle to read technical mold books. They ask for clear and easy material, and this book addresses those needs. Our approach is to use humor and pictures to help you understand the lessons quickly. We do not shy away from humorous portrayals of contractors and doctors who make people much worse. We want you to see quickly what will hurt you and your loved ones, and what will help.

- Is someone you love struggling with their behavior, mood or learning?
- Does someone in your family have allergies or asthma?
- Is their current treatment failing?
- Are you exposed to musty smells or visible mold?
- Is a family member exposed to a musty school or workplace?

The EPA reports 30% of USA structures have mold. Ten percent of USA homes leak each year, which are not dried up within 48 hours. After this time period, leaks start creating mold. But even new construction is not mold-free. Some new construction is built with moist wood and dry wall, which creates mold behind the paint.

Indoor mold is routinely present in many homes, schools, stores and other buildings. This hidden mold produces toxic chemicals on its spores that are harmful to adults and children in over 200 possible ways. Yet, because indoor mold illness is virtually absent from medical training, sincere physicians are unable to diagnose it.

Ignoring this common health threat can undermine your life, your child's life and others you love. Reading this book might help save lives. Perhaps the life you save might be your own.

Table of Contents

Home Cleaning and Vacuums 1

Mold Toxins in the Air Hurt People 3

The Effect of Indoor Mold on the Brain 4

Attics, Crawlspaces & Basements 9

Maintenance Insanity 11

The "Perfectly Fine" Filter 13

Greens are Good for Baby 15

Wacko Mold Cleaning Solutions 17

Troublesome Storage Locations and Containers 19

Carpeting and Special Rugs 21

Moving Moldy Materials 23

Happy with Mold: The Loss of Insight 25

Covering Up Mold 27

Mold and Your Head 29

The Impact of Mold Chemicals on Cognition, Emotions and Personality . . 30

Never be Surprised That Your Brain is so Sensitive 31

Musty Smells and Visible Mold 33

Summer Health 35

The Dirty Little August Secret 37

School Opens & Child Eagerness Falls 39

Problems that Come and Go 41

Child Complaints 43

Silly Mold Testing 45

More on Your New Best Friend: Filters 47

Mold as a Casual Curiosity: Losing Your Insight. 49

Most Physicians Have No Mold Toxin Training. 51

Anxiety, Depression, Agitation and ADHD 53

New Problems with a New Home, School or Job 55

Vague Cloudy Medical Diagnoses for Mold Illness 57

Allergy Trouble is NOT Mold Toxin Exposure 59

Indoor Mold: A Caring Physician is Not Enough. 61

Alternative Medicine Does Not Get It Either. 63

Mold Illness Hurts Relationships 64

An Indoor Mold or Biotoxin Symptom Checklist. 65

A Biotoxin Mold Checklist 67

Mold Toxin Use in War: More Than a Runny Nose 69

Bee Feces and Toxic Yellow Rain 69

Do Mold War Toxins Relate to You? 70

Mold Toxins Given as Cancer Treatment 71

Need Good Remediation? Become Governor! 73

You Know You Have the Wrong Remediator When... 75

Humidity Meters: A Cheap Way to Test the Waters. 76

Buying a Portable Small Humidity Meter 76

Keeping Humidity Healthy 77

Training Your Eyes to Discern Indoor Mold in Sixty Seconds. 79

Mold That is Obvious to Anyone Who is Sober 79

Powerful Lessons from Finland 85

Laboratory Testing for Mold Symptoms 87

Go Beyond Simple Allergy Labs With a Small Taste of Special Mold Labs ... 87

Melanocyte Stimulating Hormone (MSH) ... 88

MSH's Massive Role in the Body ... 89

Testing MSH ... 91

Does MSH Replacement Exist? ... 92

Leptin and Obesity ... 93

Mold with Lyme Disease or Other Infections Routinely Missed ... 94

VIP – A Powerful New Body Substance Routinely Ignored ... 95

A Small Sample of VIP References for Your Physician ... 96

The Miracle of Thermal Cameras – Why Every "Mold Expert" Must Use Them ... 97

Laser Particle Counters—Required for a Professional Remediation ... 99

A Real World Laser Particle Success Story ... 100

Blind Insurance Companies ... 101

Water-Soaked Walls: Some Basics to Save You ... 101

What is a Healthy Humidity Level? ... 102

MERV 11 Filters ... 103

The Rosen $25.00 HEPA "Machine" ... 107

Air Handler Filter Slots ... 108

Portable HEPA Machines ... 109

Comparing Filters in Common Air Filtering Devices ... 110

How To Change An Air Filter Without Filling Your Home With Mold Toxins ... 111

The Inexpensive N95 Mask Made Super Simple ... 114

N95 Mask Markings Made Easy ... 116

Common Junk Air Filters: How to Make a Duct Cleaning Company Wealthy ... 117

Handling Musty Moldy Books ... 118

What Do Mold Labs See: A Sixty Second Introduction ... 120

Basic Spore Images Used to Identify Molds 121

Black Mold Spores 124

Just Because a Mold Has No Toxins Does Not Make It Healthy 125

Dangerous Stachybotyrs or "Black Mold" 126

Powerful Mold Chemicals with Weird Names 127

The Stachy or Black Mold Fetish: Missing Other Molds 128

Additional Important Blood Testing Labs 129

Myelin Basic Protein 129

Anticardiolipin (IgA, IgG & IgM) 129

Antigliadin Antibodies 130

ANA with Reflex 130

Homocysteine 130

IgE 130

Epstein Barr Panel 131

Lab Tests Done By Quest Labs 131

VEGF – A Critical Hormone Associated with Fatigue, Aches and Concentration. 131

MMP-9 132

Complement 3a or C3a 132

Future Blood Lab Research 133

Binders, Binders and More Mold Toxin Binders 133

New Home and Building Denaturing Agents 135

Increasing the Bodies Ability to Remove Biotoxins 135

Diseases and the Clothing They Wear 136

Other Sample Mold Books by Drs. Rosen and Schaller 138

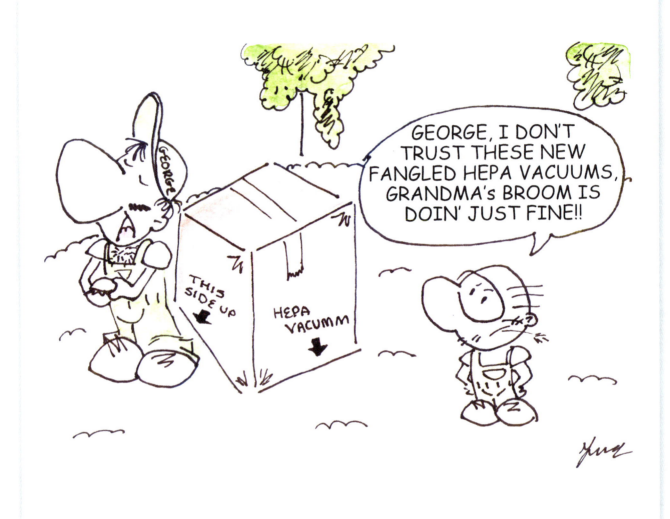

Home Cleaning and Vacuums

The guys in this first cartoon do not trust a HEPA vacuum, because it is more complicated than a broom. They feel a broom has worked for centuries. Why do they need a HEPA anything? Their ancestors survived to be thirty years old without one.

Modern homes are usually tightly sealed to be more energy-efficient. Even little water leaks that last only a few days can grow deadly molds and mold toxins. Just think of the mold toxin which makes the drug penicillin, which is antibiotic, and you are the bacteria.

One way to remove mold spores and toxins from your home is with a good vacuum that has a HEPA filter. All good new models have them. Do not use a model that requires you to shake the container to remove the dirt. You will shake billions of mold spores into the air!

What happens if you use a regular vacuum to clean up invisible mold spores on your carpet? You shoot them up into the air to fall all over your home, your loved ones and yourself.

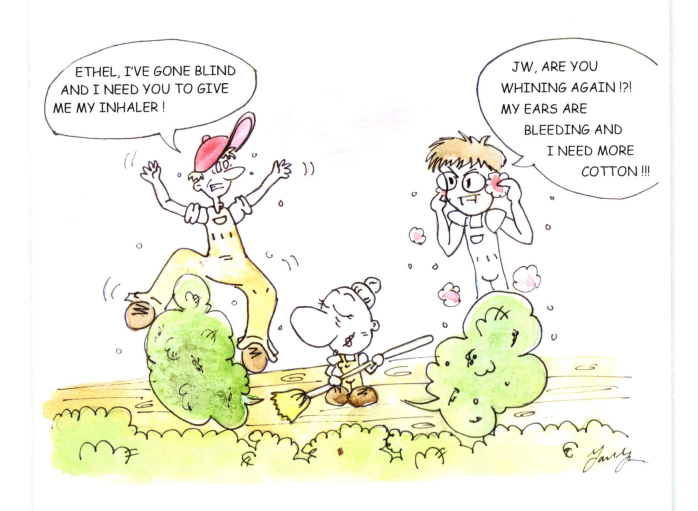

Mold Toxins in the Air Hurt People

Ethel is using a broom on the floor. It could just as easily be a regular vacuum without the ability to remove very fine dust. Mold toxins will stick to this very fine dust, and many older vacuums without HEPA filters will not properly clean contaminated dust particles.

In this cartoon, the guys are complaining of shortness of breath and bleeding ears. While mold toxins can increase asthma, the bizarre bleeding is rare.

The next three pages list some of the common symptoms of indoor mold exposure. Some people will only have a few of these problems.

The Effect of Indoor Mold on the Brain

Decreased attention

Increased risk taking

Lateness • Poor empathy

Poor boundary awareness

Increased narcissism

Poor organization

Poor stress coping

Abnormal reflexes

Serotonin changes

EEG abnormalities

Poor memory

Disorientation

Dead creativity

Vocal or Motor Tics

Seizures • Obsessive

Headaches • Immaturity

Decreased speech smoothness

Scarring of Brain seen on MRI's

Trouble with quick mental tasks

Child developmental milestone delays

Decreased productivity

Trouble speaking fast

Irritability • Impulsivity

Mood swings • Mania

Trouble finding words

Trouble concentrating

Depression • Anxiety

Trouble learning

Forgetfulness

Eccentric personality

Strokes • Trembling

Poor insight into illness

Increased verbal fighting

Unable to process trauma

Drug abuse • Panic Attacks

Increased alcohol consumption

Spacey • Rigidity • Poor insight

Edema or swelling in the brain

Abnormal PET and SPECT scans

Highly sensitive to interpersonal problems

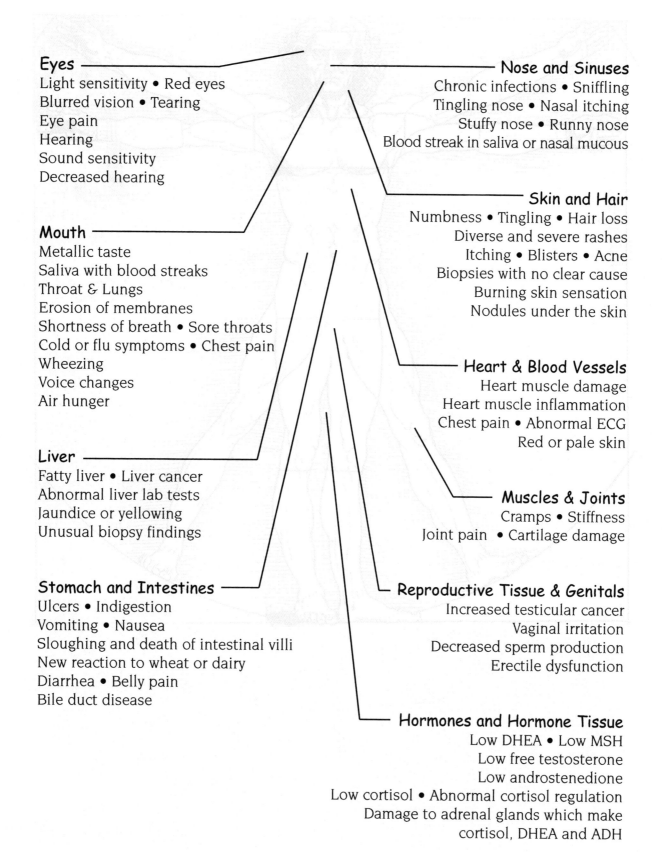

Eyes
Light sensitivity • Red eyes
Blurred vision • Tearing
Eye pain
Hearing
Sound sensitivity
Decreased hearing

Mouth
Metallic taste
Saliva with blood streaks
Throat & Lungs
Erosion of membranes
Shortness of breath • Sore throats
Cold or flu symptoms • Chest pain
Wheezing
Voice changes
Air hunger

Liver
Fatty liver • Liver cancer
Abnormal liver lab tests
Jaundice or yellowing
Unusual biopsy findings

Stomach and Intestines
Ulcers • Indigestion
Vomiting • Nausea
Sloughing and death of intestinal villi
New reaction to wheat or dairy
Diarrhea • Belly pain
Bile duct disease

Nose and Sinuses
Chronic infections • Sniffling
Tingling nose • Nasal itching
Stuffy nose • Runny nose
Blood streak in saliva or nasal mucous

Skin and Hair
Numbness • Tingling • Hair loss
Diverse and severe rashes
Itching • Blisters • Acne
Biopsies with no clear cause
Burning skin sensation
Nodules under the skin

Heart & Blood Vessels
Heart muscle damage
Heart muscle inflammation
Chest pain • Abnormal ECG
Red or pale skin

Muscles & Joints
Cramps • Stiffness
Joint pain • Cartilage damage

Reproductive Tissue & Genitals
Increased testicular cancer
Vaginal irritation
Decreased sperm production
Erectile dysfunction

Hormones and Hormone Tissue
Low DHEA • Low MSH
Low free testosterone
Low androstenedione
Low cortisol • Abnormal cortisol regulation
Damage to adrenal glands which make cortisol, DHEA and ADH

Overall Body

Fatigue
Weakness
Malaise
Eccentric weight gain
Occasionally eccentric thinness
Bizarre pain
Ice pick pain
Lightning bolt pain
New chemical sensitivity
Spinning sensation or dizziness
Increased thirst
Frequent urination
Shocking sensation
Sweats
Temperature variation
Appetite swings
Easy bleeding or bruising
Swelling
Trouble walking or running easily
Reduced coordination
Rapid pulse
Low temperature
Jerky movements
Abnormal blood pressure (low or high)
Fever
Chills
Increased tumors

Which of the Signs and Symptoms on the Previous Pages Apply to You?

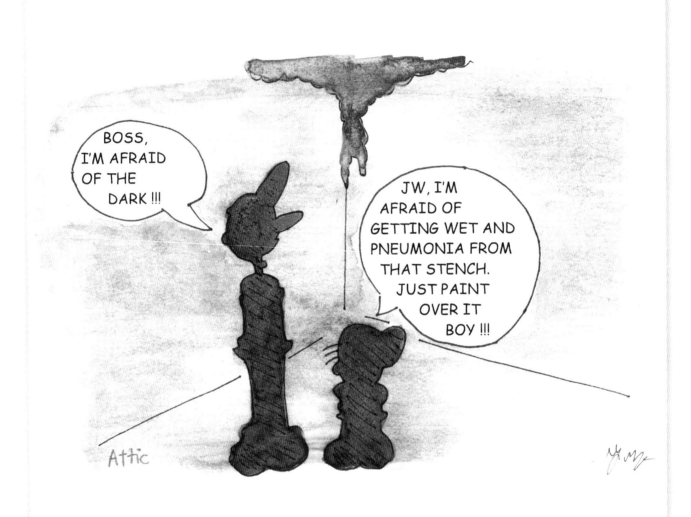

Attics, Crawlspaces & Basements

In many suspense films, the main character is walking down dark stairs or going up into an attic with spider webs. You just know the surprise in the dark is not going to be a birthday party. In the same way, basements and attics are prime mold breeding grounds that make them scary.

Basements and crawl spaces often have moisture from leaks or condensation on the walls and floors. If the humidity is above 65%, you will likely start making Aspergillus or Penicillium. Most of these species are not healthy molds.

Attics are frequently hot and humid. Roof leaks often start by water entering the attic and hitting drywall, cardboard storage boxes, paper insulation, plywood and dust.

In the cartoon, the guys see visible mold. According to the Environmental Protection Agency (EPA), if you see or smell mold, it has to be removed. The indoor mold you see is always assumed to be toxic, and what you smell is mold poop. Painting over it is insanity, but commonly done. Why? Fixing moldy or musty areas in a home, school or business is not as easy as a little paint.

Bubba worries about getting "pneumonia." In a wet environment, many types of bacteria can grow. Some types make toxins.

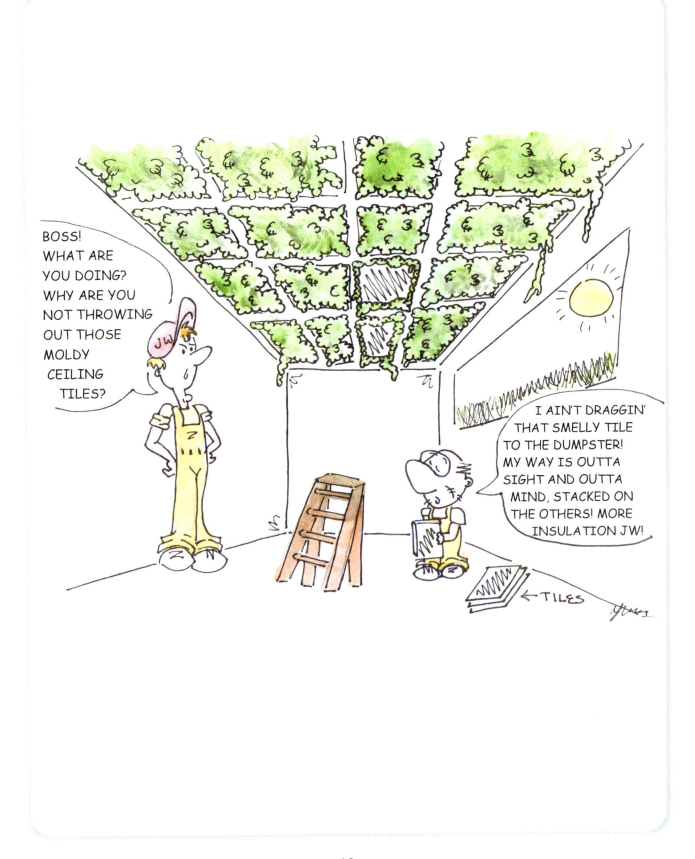

Maintenance Insanity

Last week, a maintenance man took an air filter out of my ceiling and put it on the floor. He then carried it out without first putting it in a bag – dropping billions of mold spores as he walked.

Maintenance workers have no mold training. No one offers it to them. As a result, people suffer in schools, buildings and apartment complexes.

This cartoon shows a common and serious error made by maintenance staff. Water drips onto the ceiling tiles and grows mold. The watermarks and discoloration are ugly, so the tiles are replaced. Are they thrown out?

No. The moldy ceiling tiles are pushed on top of other tiles and a collection of moldy tiles contaminates the entire ceiling.

American society knows nothing about basic school, business or home health. Indoor mold releases chemicals that cause severe inflammation of many possible body organs, while these toxins also lower insight. Sincere maintenance people simply do not realize the severe consequences of their actions.

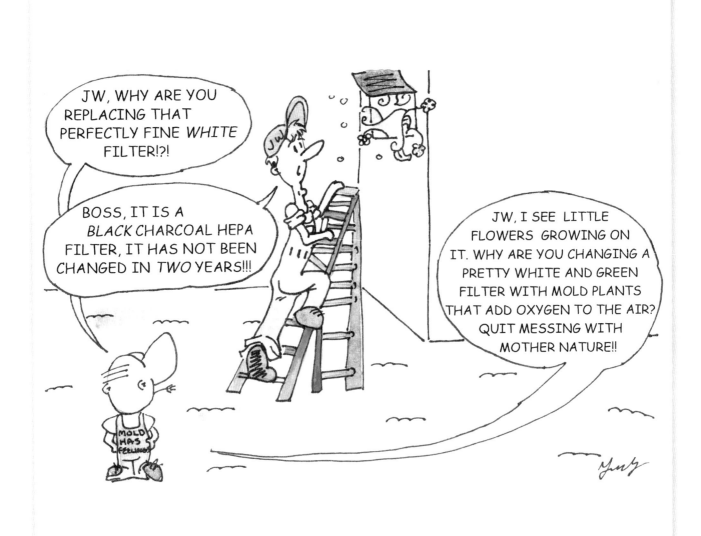

The "Perfectly Fine" Filter

Air conditioning companies have more gimmicks than used car salesmen. These include metal electrostatic air filters or permanent filters. You never want to save toxic mold dust inside a metal filter. You do not want to be exposed to toxins when cleaning a permanent filter. Think of filters like toilet tissue. Would you clean toilet tissue? Filters should be replaced every month in a moldy or dusty home, or two months in a very clean home.

Air conditioning workers have told us that business and home filters they replaced are often caked with dust — perfect mold food. Obviously, these overloaded filters are probably just preventing airflow. This will cause dirt build up on the filter — creating mold heaven.

The best filters are MERV 11 disposable filters and are available at Home Depot, Lowe's, Wal-Mart and at www.filters-now.com. The latter company can make any size you want and has hundreds of sizes in stock. The MERV 11 rating means it will catch fine dust particles and the smallest mold spores. You will dust less and never need to clean out your AC ducts when you use MERV 11 filters.

Do not get a MERV 15 since that requires a very powerful AC fan motor and is not needed. You do not need to filter electrons!

Some stores offer a very thin charcoal filter that will remove the gases coming off new carpets, computers, TV screens and mold. These can often be used on top of the Merv 11 filters.

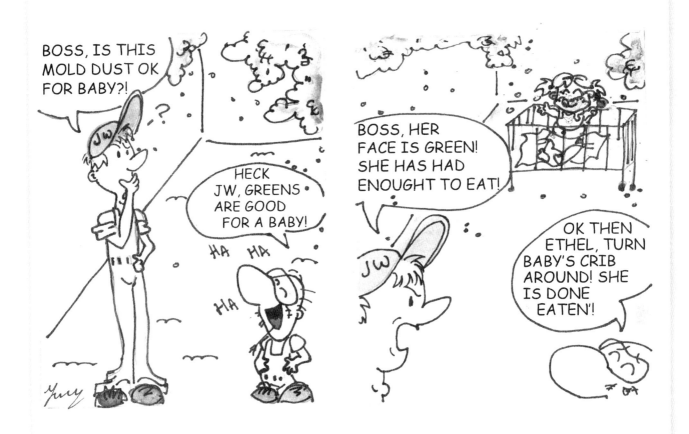

Greens are Good for Baby

There is simply no "safe" level of mold toxin. Most Americans are casual about mold because they do not know it causes over two hundred medical problems and can kill. It increases clotting in the blood stream that causes heart attacks and strokes. Mold toxins also lower natural killer cells, the cells you use to fight cancer. So you are at an increased risk of getting cancer.

Children and the elderly are particularly at risk for bodily injury from molds. Here we see a toddler that is exposed in a home. The toddler cannot tell you if he or she feels badly. But they might be harder to soothe, have colic or develop more slowly. Just recall, as many as 30% of US structures have mold — that means millions of children and elderly are being exposed.

This cartoon also shows the tremendous shortsightedness about indoor mold. Some molds in homes have toxins that have been used in warfare, and are aggressively controlled by the USDA to keep them out of the foods we eat. Many brilliant people treat mold like a spice, when it is more like anthrax.

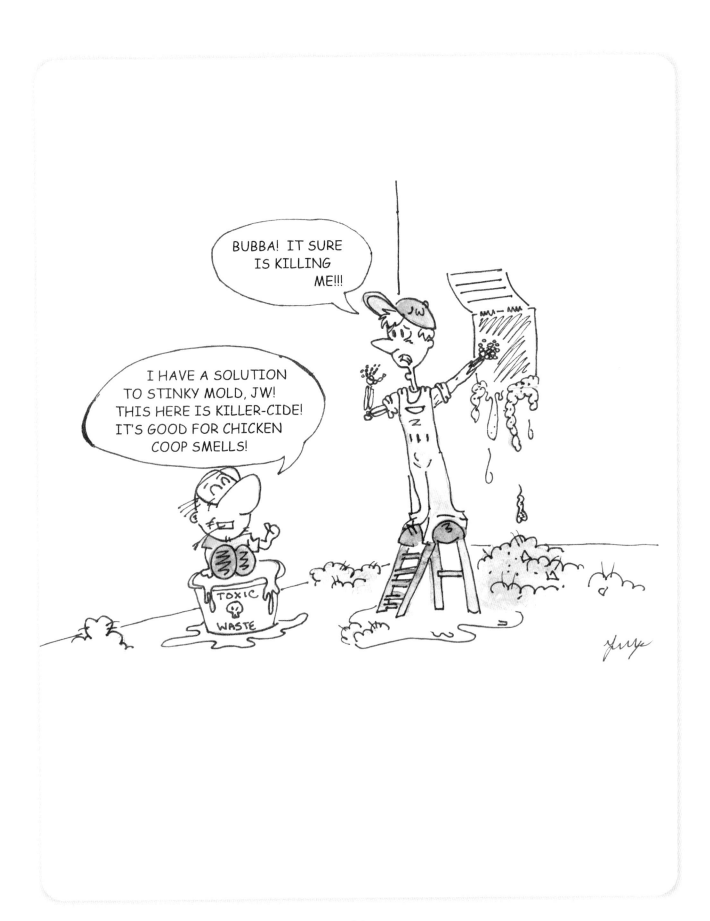

Wacko Mold Cleaning Solutions

There is no EPA approved chemical to spray into moldy or dusty air conditioning ducts. A bleach solution may kill loose spores and the top spores in a mound of mold, but it will not penetrate dust and enter the bottom of a mold mound. Many AC cleaning and maintenance companies use alkaline cleaners to spray in air handlers and other duct handlers. This is a very strong cleaner and may weaken some synthetic and natural materials, but it does kill bacteria and mold.

Be alert to what is being sprayed in your home ducts. You will be breathing this chemical. Some AC cleaning companies use very toxic chemicals that kill mold, but will also hurt your lungs and make you ill.

Consider looking on their bottle or getting the name of the cleaner before they come. Look it up on the Internet or call your local poison control center with the name of the chemical.

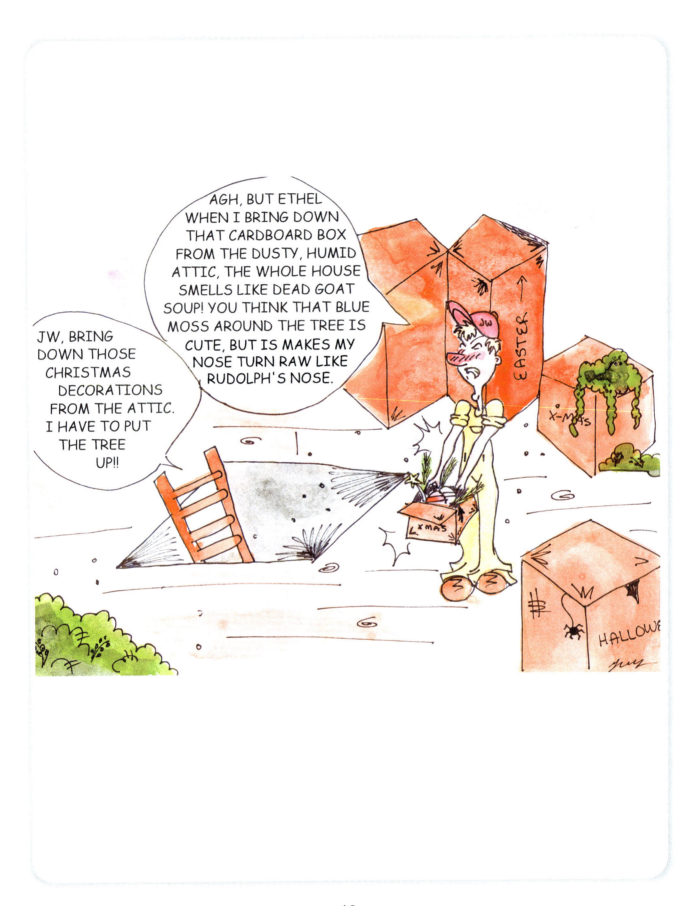

Troublesome Storage Locations and Containers

The most common storage places in a home are the attic, basement, garage and crawlspace. Any of these can have high humidity or water. The high humidity and water will grow common toxic molds. If your storage container is clear strong plastic, the mold cannot grow on it. If you use cardboard boxes for storage, you are laying out a Thanksgiving Day feast for mold.

Use strong plastic containers to store your materials. The thin and weak ones crack easily and have a poor seal, and then you will have water and humidity inside the container. We do not recommend the routine use of mothballs due to toxic fumes. Instead, we suggest preserving materials in containers with a slight mist of alcohol-based Lysol, or adding an open bag of Borax. Either should prevent any mold growth. Test each on a non-critical piece of what is being stored, to confirm it will not damage it.

A routine problem is that once you have mold growth in a basement, garage or attic, you can easily spread it. How?

- You carry a container coated with mold to another room inside your house.
- You allow air in a moldy area like a moist garage or attic to be sucked into the rest of the home.

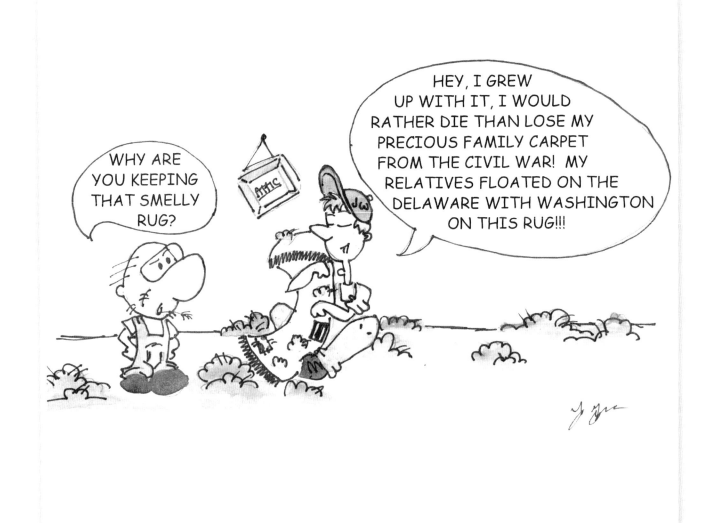

Carpeting and Special Rugs

During a remediation job at a school, we found that we could not reduce the mold spores to any tolerable level. Finally, we told the school officials that the old rugs, which had been moist from leaks over a ten-year period had to go, period.

They understood. The bookcases and AC intake vents were covered. We used filtering masks from Home Depot. The classrooms were sealed with simple plastic sheets over the doors so spores did not fly all over the school. We sprayed the surface of the carpet with some Sklar disinfectant lightly misted on top, cut and rolled up the carpet pieces, and tossed them out the window. No spores were going to fly around on us! We also had two strong fans sending all the dust and loose spores out the window. And we worked with high quality air filtering machines, called air scrubbers.

Some special oriental rugs can be saved with special cleaning, dry cleaning and other interventions. But please try not to save regular carpeting that most likely contains mold.

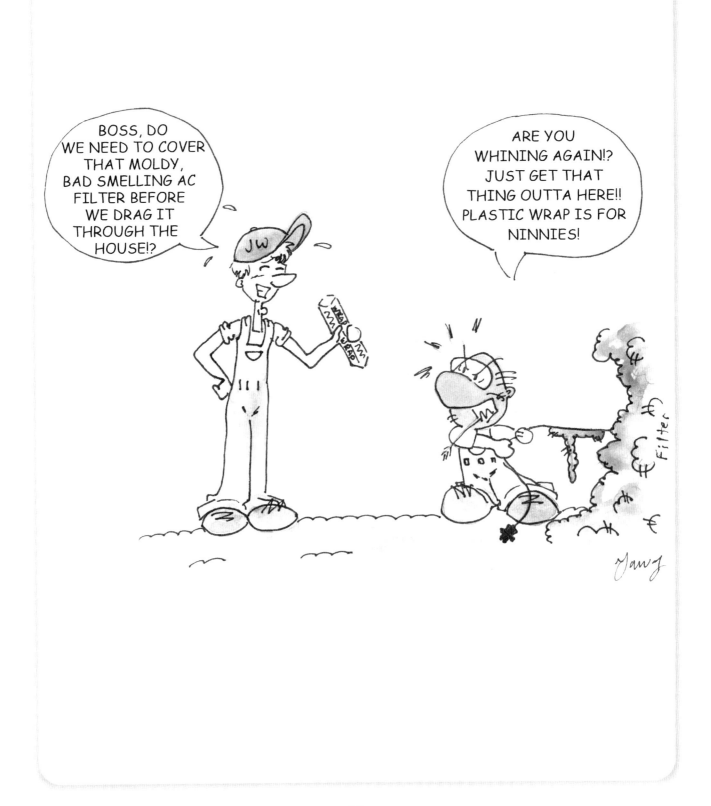

Moving Moldy Materials

In this cartoon, the boss thinks that it is silly to seal a moldy article before carrying it through the home. Typically, most people and most contractors carry moldy dry wall, moldy boards, moldy plywood and moldy boxes through homes, schools and businesses. They disburse billions of spores inside as they walk to the exit.

Any dirty air filter or moldy item has to be sealed in a strong plastic bag or plastic sheeting before it is moved. It is very unwise to ignore this basic mold principle, but most workers you hire will not seal materials they remove.

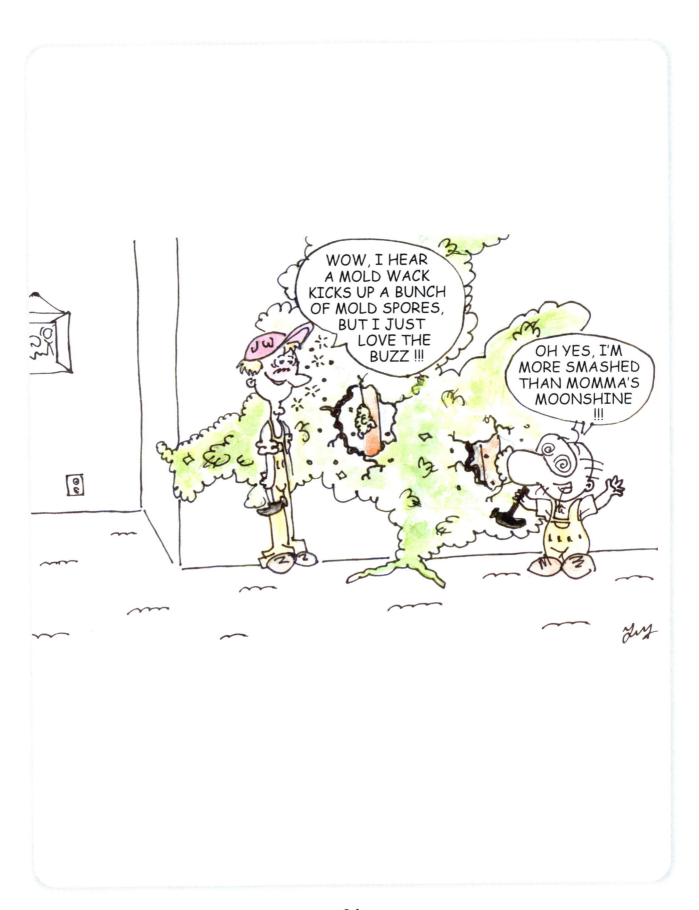

Happy with Mold: The Loss of Insight

Some people do not care about indoor mold illness. They do not appreciate that mold toxins increase many inflammation chemicals, which clot the blood and can alter your mood. Mold toxins also commonly alter a wide range of hormones, some of which are important but not routinely tested.

We have talked to thousands about indoor mold problems, and some are just too far-gone to realize their minds are already being affected by mold. They are standing in quicksand and simply cannot be bothered.

In this cartoon, we see Bubba and JW have no sense of the danger of mold.

Our appeal would be to take seriously any mold you see or smell, or which might be present in your homes or buildings due to past or present leaks, or other types of water exposure.

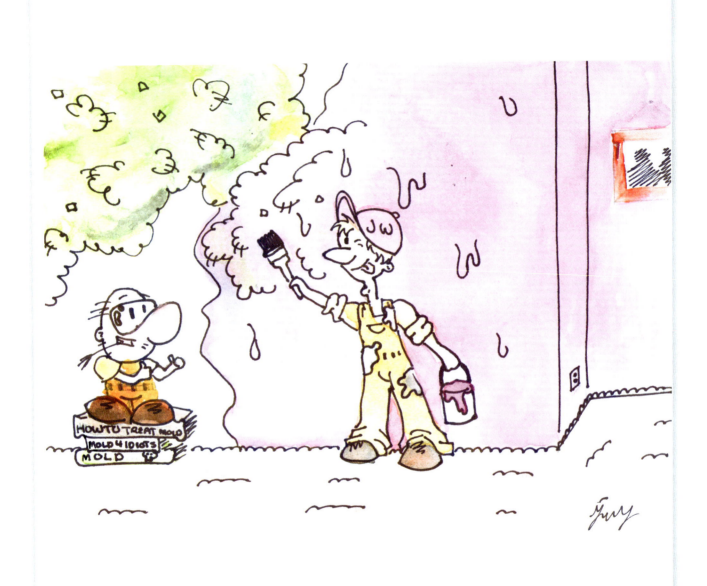

Covering Up Mold

Many homeowners with a mold problem will not spend the money to fix the problem. They will hide it and sell their home. Most homes can be remediated and fixed for a modest cost, but it would be good for you to buy Gary Rosen's **Mold Remediation and Mold Toxins: What You Need to Know Before Hiring a Remediator** from www.Mold-Free.org. He is a master builder, a veteran mold remediator and a scientist who understands the science of mold. If you do not know the basics, you cannot evaluate the solutions suggested.

In this cartoon, we see someone knowingly painting over a mold patch. So if you are buying a property, have a smart tester do some air collection samples. Do not use simple Petri dishes, since they always show an unreliable positive. Generally, if problem levels of mold are hiding in a wall or ceiling behind paint, it will show up in an air test. The most common air test is the use of a Zefon Air-O-Cell cartridge. It is really a simple device. The tester attaches this plastic cartridge to a suction machine for 5-10 minutes in a suspect room, with the cartridge a foot off the ground to catch heavy types of spores. Then they mail it off to a testing laboratory, where a lab tech counts the mold spores they see under a microscope.

Commonly, ignorant mold testers report a home has no mold if it has the same number of spores as an outside sample. This is nonsense. If your home has MERV 11 filters in its AC filtering system, then a mold-free home should have a fraction of the mold found in the outside air. Any mold inspector who says a home, school or business is "clean" when the indoor mold levels are the same as outdoor levels — is ignorant.

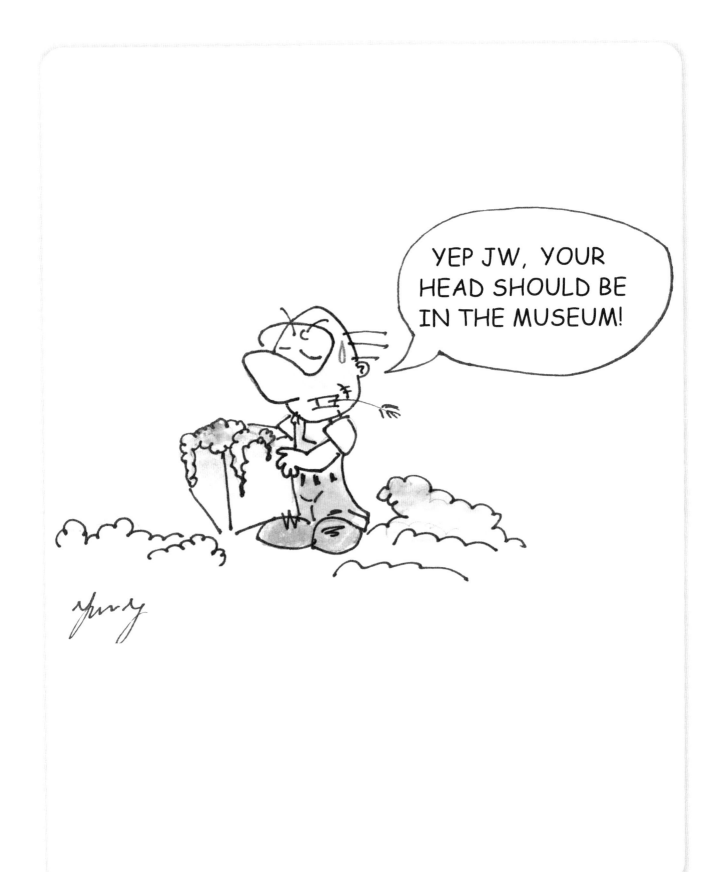

Mold and Your Head

Many physicians are completely blind to the neurological and psychological symptoms of mold. Physicians only receive about two hours of mold education in medical school and residency. Why would they diagnose what they have never been trained to see?

We know contractors who have not been trained in smart mold practices. They do not follow wise mold protection techniques. So they end up foggy, thinking slowly, or on edge.

Mold toxins can occasionally cause autoimmunity. For example, your immune system attacks your own nerves.

Here is a small sample of mold toxin effects to the brain:

- Headaches
- Poor memory
- Trouble concentrating
- Trouble learning
- Trouble finding words
- Disorientation
- Trouble speaking fast
- Slow thinking
- Slow comprehension
- Trouble following rapid speech
- PET and SPECT scans show abnormalities
- Seizures
- Trembling
- Vocal or motor tics
- Serotonin changes
- Abnormal reflexes
- Strokes
- Edema or swelling in the brain
- Scarring of brain seen on MRI's
- EEG abnormalities

The Impact of Mold Chemicals on Cognition, Emotions and Personality

- Mood swings
- Mania
- Irritability
- Impulsivity
- Increased risk taking
- Decreased speech smoothness
- Poor stress coping
- Increased verbal fighting
- Lateness
- Poor empathy
- Poor boundary awareness
- Immaturity
- Spacey
- Rigidity
- Poor insight
- Poor insight into illness
- Decreased productivity
- Unable to process trauma or interpersonal pain
- Increased narcissism
- Forgetfulness
- Poorly organized or obsessively organized
- Dead creativity
- Depression
- Anxiety
- Panic attacks
- Decreased attention
- Eccentric personality
- A delay in a child's developmental milestones
- Increased alcohol consumption or increased drug use

Never be Surprised That Your Brain is so Sensitive

Important Personality Changes

Some physicians do not appreciate that the brain is the most sensitive organ in the body. It is the most sensitive to blood chemistry changes. They know that the brain will die in minutes without oxygen or sugar, but do not realize that many chemicals will negatively affect the brain. These common body chemicals alter personality, mood, memory and concentration.

One group of chemicals that alter thinking and mood are hundreds of biological chemicals made by your own body or made by other living organisms. Some increase your stroke and heart attack risk. Mold toxins are biologically active chemicals made by mold which can cause inflammation in your blood and increase your risk for blood clots.

In light of the seriousness of mold exposure, we are surprised to see most patients never receive any yearly evaluation of their inflammation and clotting system.

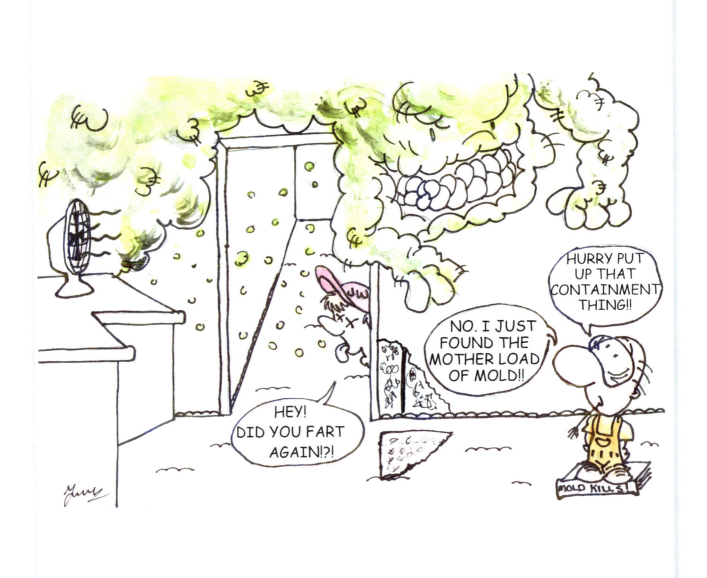

Musty Smells and Visible Mold

In this cartoon, JW and Bubba smell and see mold. If you are able to do either in your home, school, workplace or place of worship, you are being exposed to mold toxins.

Someone can do all the testing they want, but according to the EPA, mold that is emitting an odor or is visible, must be removed.

In this cartoon, the guys did not prepare the room to prevent mold release when opening a moist wall cavity. So as soon as they took off a piece of drywall with mold, their fan blew spores everywhere. Also, they did not hang plastic to keep the spores contained, nor did they use a mask or skin protection. Mold toxins can be inhaled, swallowed or can pass directly through uncovered skin, so the remediators and you will all become ill.

If this is your home, school or workplace, these guys have just contaminated the entire structure, because the air ducts will carry the spores all over the building. Spores will also settle on the ground and be carried on shoes at a rate that depends on the traffic.

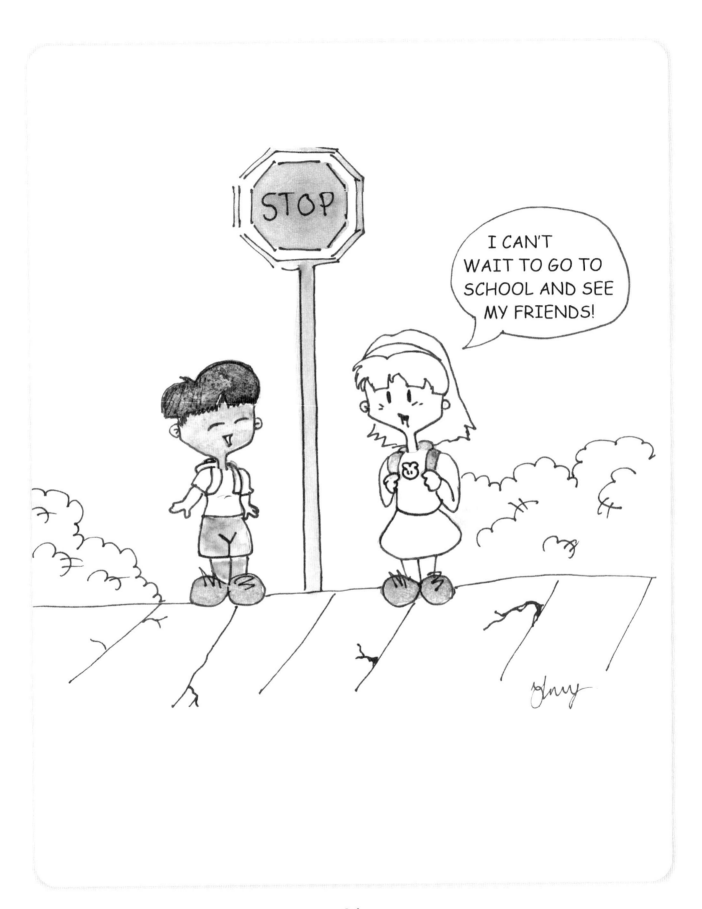

Summer Health

Many children have better moods and clearer thinking while away from a sick school building, especially during the summer months.

Some youth do not notice their school affects them negatively. So during the summer they start to fantasize about seeing their school friends.

Unfortunately, many schools have been made with cheap AC systems that are too costly to run or maintain. So a contractor gets a contract to build a school because he has the lowest price, but he also installs a cheap and poor quality HVAC system that will not control humidity and mold. The excess mold slowly destroys the health of the students.

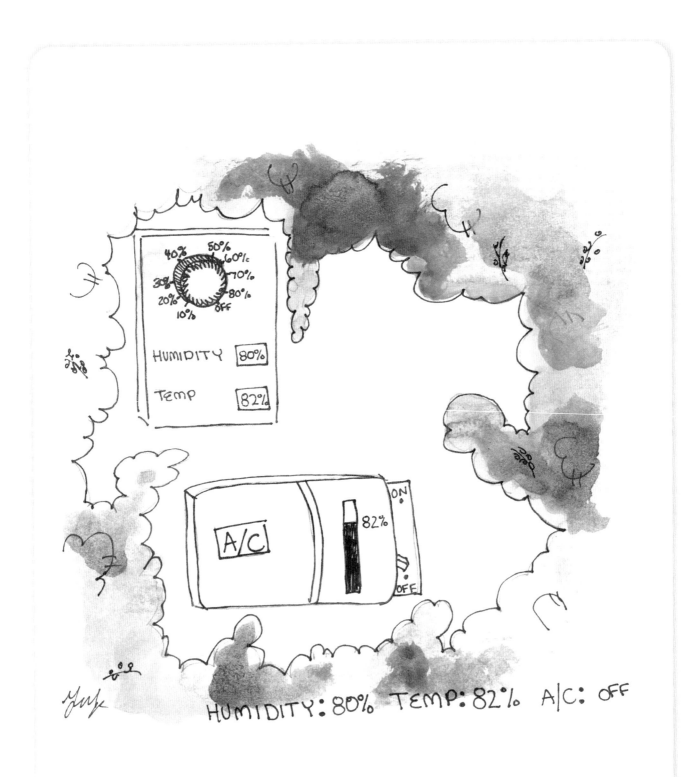

The Dirty Little August Secret

When schools are closed for the summer, the administration has the AC turned off to save money. The result is that the temperature and the humidity skyrocket and the school becomes a greenhouse. The first "plants" to grow in this greenhouse are molds.

They grow in the ceilings. They grow on the books. They grow on the walls and inside the venting system.

When the school year starts, and the air conditioning is turned on, the mold spores and dust with mold toxins will be dispersed all over the school.

Humidity over 65% runs the risk of growing indoor mold.

If a school, home or business has a power outage, such as from a fallen tree limb, a flood or a hurricane, the air conditioning system will fail. If the indoor humidity rises to 80%, you will start producing indoor mold in two days.

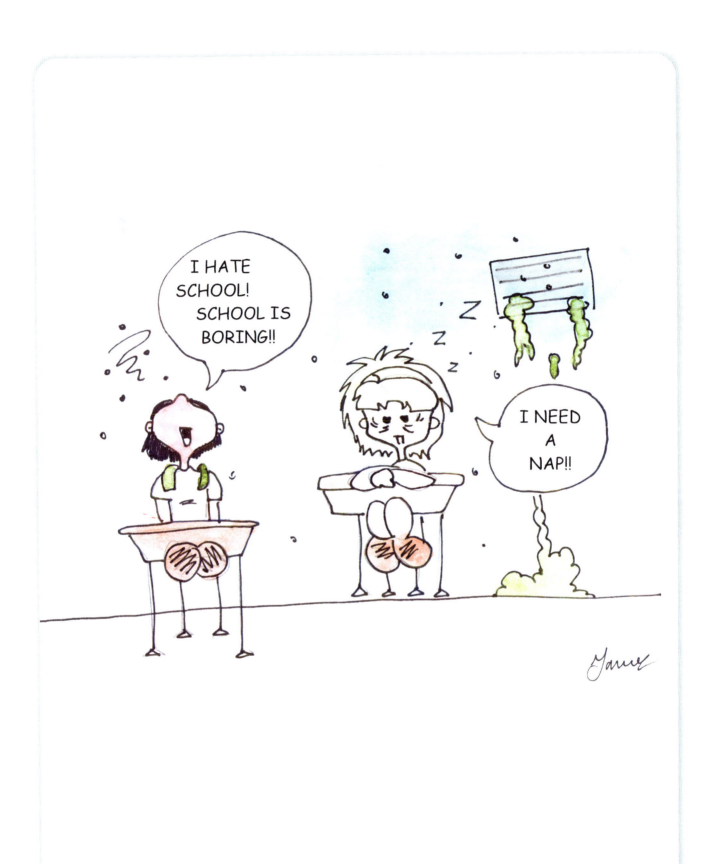

School Opens & Child Eagerness Falls

Children who are looking forward to returning to school change quickly in the presence of indoor mold. Children that had interest in science are less interested. A teacher who is slightly interesting is utterly boring, since a mold-exposed child finds most things more boring.

Children that ran for hours in the hot summer sun, are now exhausted sitting for short periods in their moldy classrooms.

If the mold is not in their class, but is in the gym or some other part of the structure, it will make its way to every room in the school through the air ducts.

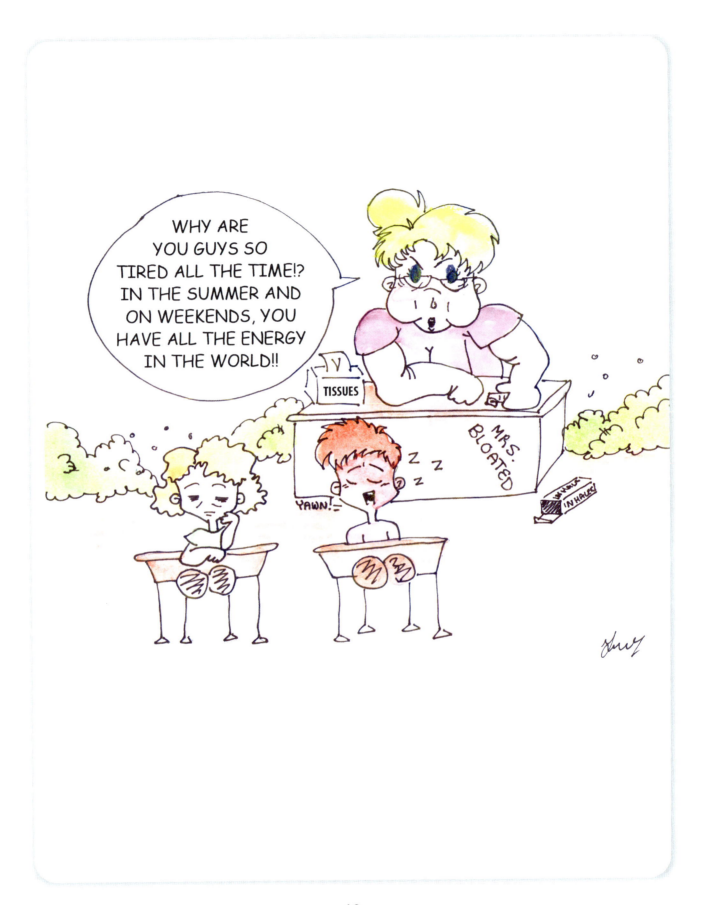

Problems that Come and Go

In this cartoon, Mrs. Bloated asks why the kids are alert and active on weekends and in the summer, but not at school. We see this in contractors with poor mold training all the time. They go into a clean house and feel fine. They enter a home with toxic forms of Aspergillus and Penicillium and feel ill. They enter a home with black mold or Stachybotrys and they are terribly ill.

Over time, a child or adult may become primed from repeated mold exposure, so that they do not get any better when they are in a mold-free home or different school. They will require mold toxin binders and other special treatments to turn off their excess inflammation. They will need special interventions to fix hormone changes routinely missed by allergists, occupational physicians, toxicologists and family doctors.

Mrs. Bloated is also affected and as the cartoon shows, she needs tissues, an inhaler, and is bloated and obese from mold toxins. We have treated patients who underwent bariatric surgery for their weight increase as a result of mold toxin exposure. Eventually, they gained back some weight due to ongoing mold exposure and possibly due to a very low MSH. The latter is melanocyte-stimulating hormone, which has twenty roles and is involved with weight control.

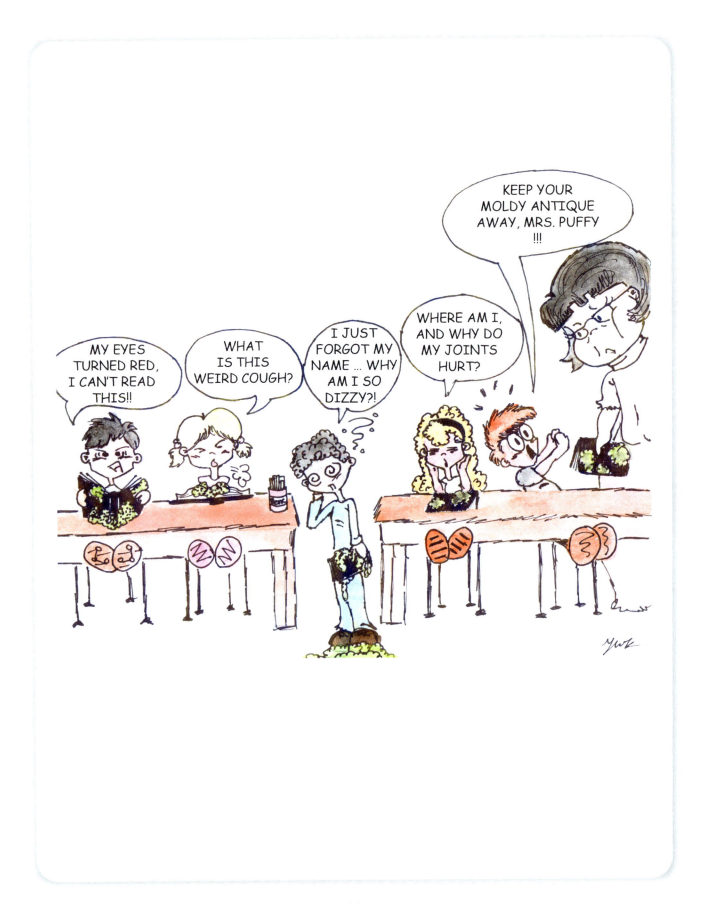

Child Complaints

This cartoon shows some common youth complaints in a moldy school or home. Adults in moldy buildings can have similar struggles. Often, they think their deficits are normal. At other times, they are entirely unaware that mold is hurting them — they have very poor insight, even if they are very smart.

The teachers and administrators at a school also often have poor insight. Many are very quick to find some character faults, parental troubles or psychological explanations for why little Johnny or Sue is acting up.

Schools are sometimes filled with pretend psychologists and psychiatrists in these situations, who toss around insulting labels for children with troubled behavior, based on a couple articles they have read. Yet many of these children have biotoxins and brain inflammation from mold or other sources, e.g., Lyme or Bartonella. In our experience, once mold is cleared up, many "bad" boys and girls suddenly become very reasonable. Their medical illness caused many of them to struggle to behave, as biotoxins and inflammation "gasoline" floated around in their veins. Once it was fixed, they were able to follow the rules.

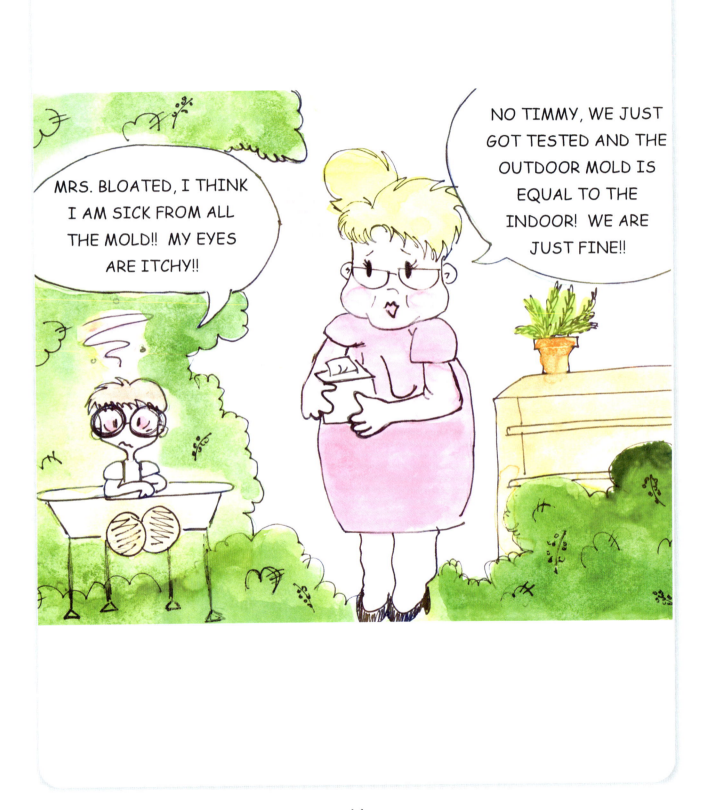

Silly Mold Testing

Mrs. Bloated explains that the school had been tested and the results showed the school was "just fine." If a business owner, builder or landlord wants to get their structure "cleared" there are plenty of poorly educated mold testers who will report that a mushroom factory is just fine!

One common mold tester error is the position that if a home, building or school has the same mold counts indoors as outdoors, then all is well. Incorrect! Indoor mold should be scrubbed from indoor air by the AC air filters and should typically be 10% or less of outdoor air levels in a healthy building. Further, indoor mold has less competition and has no UV radiation exposure, so indoor molds are more likely to make biotoxins.

In this cartoon, we hear the children report troubles with their eyes, an eccentric cough, and aches in their muscles and joints.

Notice one child is "dizzy" — which is a neurological complaint. Indeed, many youth have learning troubles and other neurological troubles related to mold.

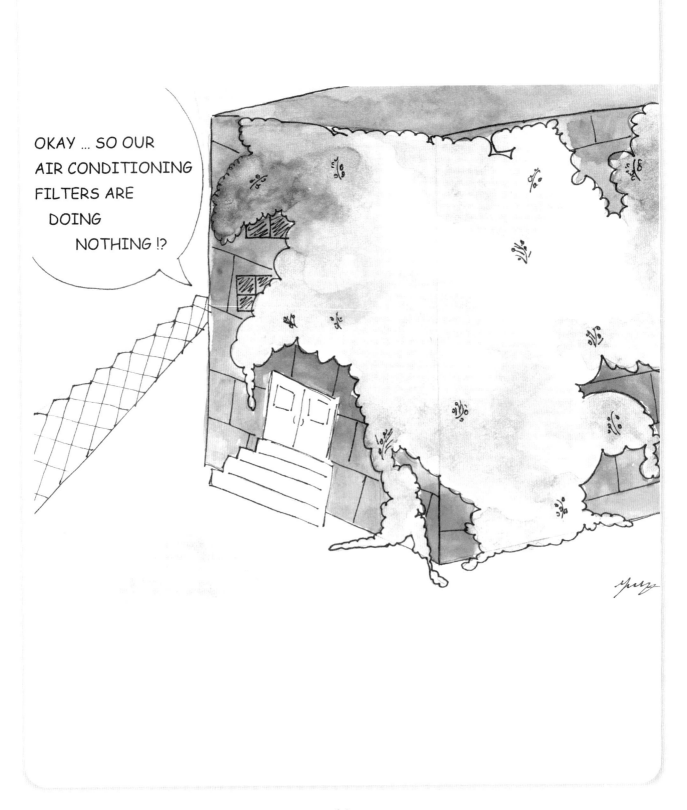

More on Your New Best Friend: Filters

Every building, home and school needs disposable MERV 11 filters that capture dust filled with mold toxins. This will end the need to clean dusty ducts and will scrub the air. No filter should ever be left in for over two months, and if filters are changed every one to two months in homes, schools and businesses, a massive amount of contaminated mold dust will be removed.

If a home or contaminated office does not have a filter on an AC unit, one cheap effective option is to purchase a couple of 20-inch box fans. Then buy some 20 inch x 20 inch MERV 11 filters and tape them to the back of the box fan. (We show pictures of how to construct this "Dr. Rosen fan" later in the book). Run the fan as much as you can. In places with toxic mold dust, these home made air scrubbers will scrub mold residues and may allow people to stay healthy. Replace the filters every 4-8 weeks.

However, be careful not to allow MERV 11 filters or portable devices to promote casualness about visible mold or mold odors. Fans cannot remove serious mold intrusion.

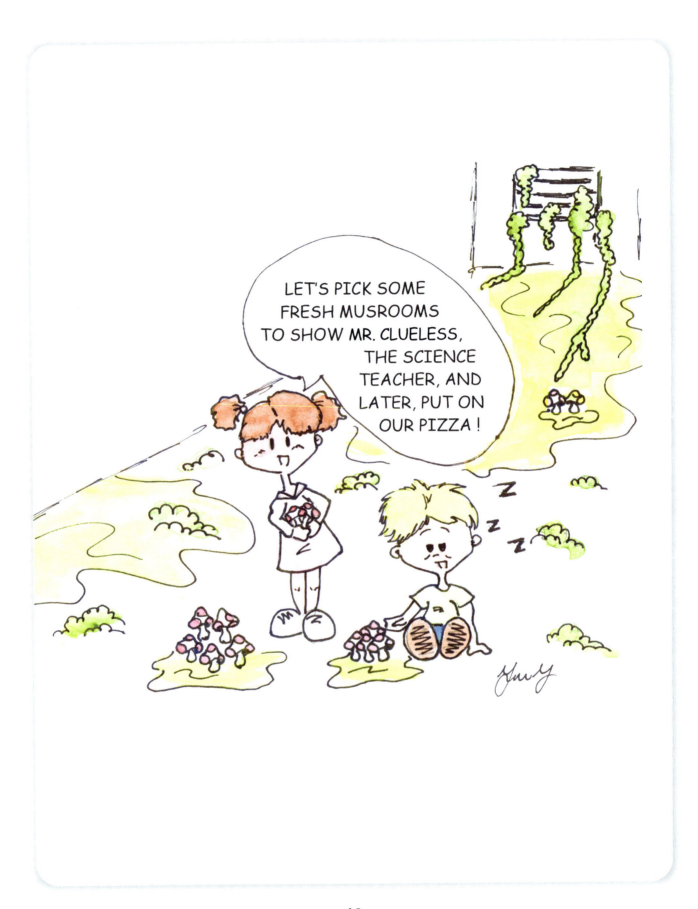

Mold as a Casual Curiosity: Losing Your Insight

Mold is able to blind you to its effects. Many mold experts say it took years for them to notice slight shifts in their attention, energy, and personality created by mold. One of the side effects of mold exposure is decreased awareness of its effects on you.

Since most Americans and their physicians do not understand the effects of mold toxins, people will wrongly diagnose your struggles, or the problems of your child and say:

- You are spacey and you have ADD or ADHD.
- You are a moody and nasty person.
- You are "lazy" and have no initiative.
- You are an addict or an alcoholic. (The abuse of substances is often an attempt to create good feelings, because one of your "feel good" hormones, MSH, is low).

Mold toxins have the ability to alter any aspect of your life. It is really just that simple. And when they alter an aspect of your life, you can assume you will be clueless about it.

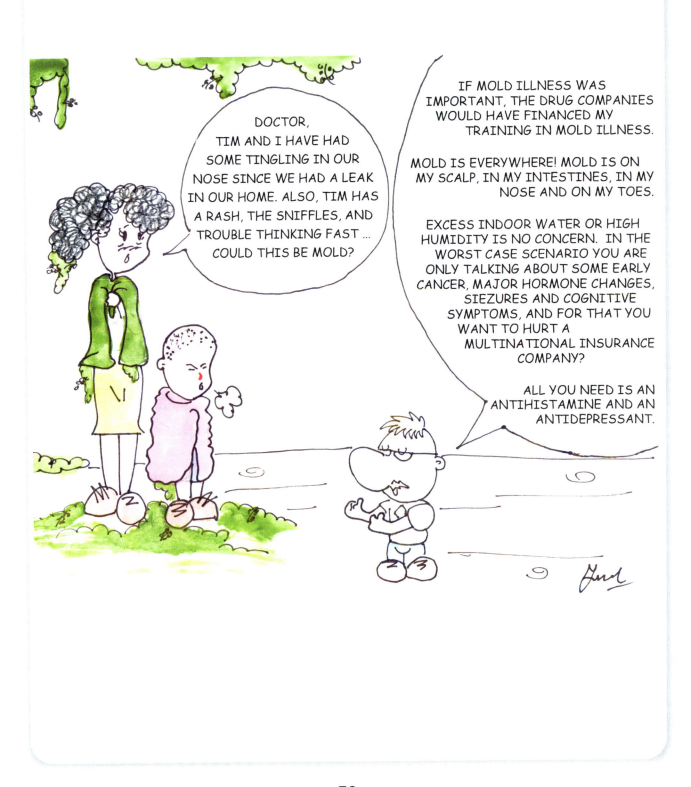

Most Physicians Have No Mold Toxin Training

I cannot speak Chinese. So when I see a Chinese article, it means nothing to me. Physicians get about two hours of mold training over nine years. So it is entirely expected most cannot "see" mold toxin effects.

Each day patients of every age are feeling mild and severe effects from mold. When they ask their physicians about these problems, physicians look to their earlier training for answers, but that training excluded mold toxins.

In this cartoon, we see a mother and her child "hand-feeding" the physician the diagnosis of mold toxin exposure, and yet he could not see it. Unfortunately, some physicians are stressed due to poor cash flow and huge malpractice insurance premiums. They are unsettled by any diagnosis outside pharmaceutical company medical knowledge. So what happens when mold is raised as a cause when all the other routine options do not fully cure? The patient is insulted, treated as a bore, and their creative thinking is seen as the reflections of a quack.

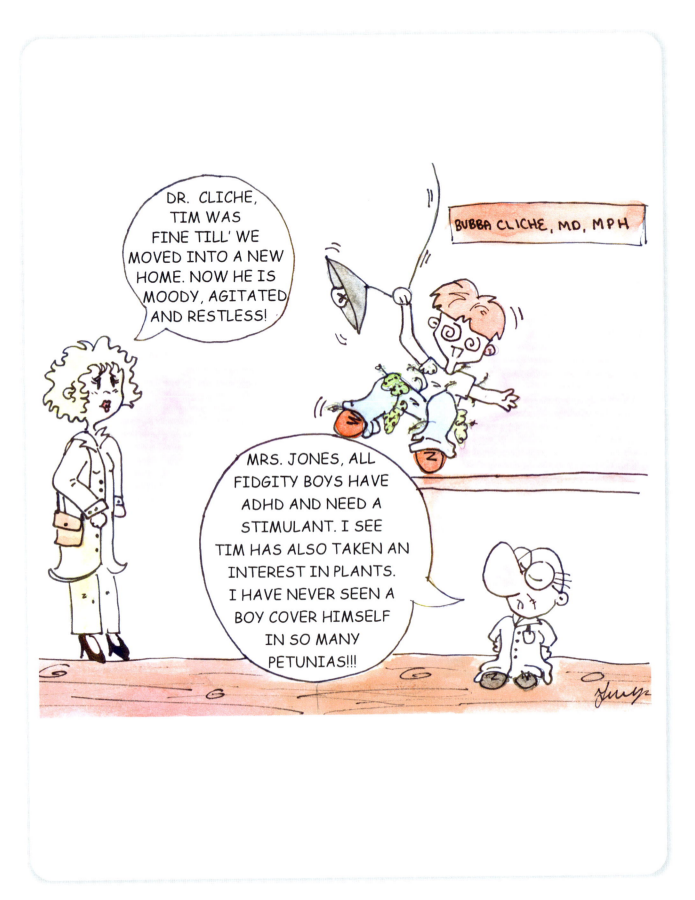

Anxiety, Depression, Agitation and ADHD

Mold causes increased body inflammation. If you could inject these inflammation chemicals into a person, they might manifest symptoms of anxiety, depression, agitation or ADHD.

While all of these disorders can be due to genetic problems, they can also be caused by hundreds of medical problems.

As a research physician and clinical child and adolescent psychiatrist, I can say that mold and tick-borne Lyme illness are the two most common medical causes for emotional problems missed by pediatricians, internists, family doctors, specialists and psychiatrists. To learn more about these issues go to:

- **Mold Warriors: Fighting America's Hidden Health Threat**. This 600-page book was written by Dr. Shoemaker, Dr. Schaller and Patti Schmidt. It can be ordered from **www.moldwarriors.com** or **Amazon.com**.
- **When Traditional Medicine Fails: Your Guide to Mold Toxins**. An easy-to-read powerful mold illness and mold remediation book by Drs. Rosen and Schaller. This book is available from **Amazon.com**.
- Dr. Schaller's 2,500 page free website, **www.personalconsult.com**, under "mold" or "Lyme disease."
- Dr. Schaller is currently writing a book on pediatric tick-borne infections with the top pediatric tick infection expert in the country. This 78 year-old expert has treated 9,000 children with tick-borne infections such as Lyme, Babesia and Bartonella.

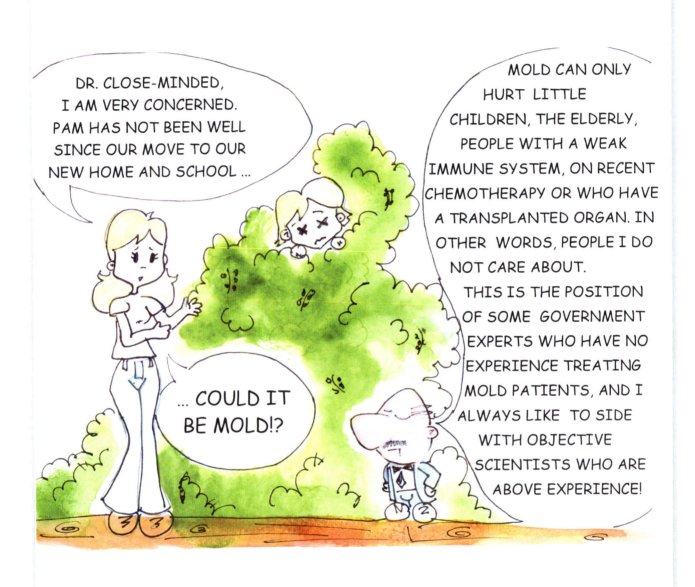

New Problems with a New Home, School or Job

This mother wisely noted a change in her child that started after a move. She does not know if it is her child's home or the school or both, but she knows something is different. She is not sure if mold is the cause, but she is considering the possibility. Because she is open to this possibility, she is far ahead of the limited knowledge of most physicians.

As the cartoon explains, mold is felt to be a problem in humans — but only as an actual infection. Mold spores are seen as a cause of chronic sinus infections, and as an invading infection in those with no functional immune system, like those with HIV infections.

However, physicians must understand that the chemicals covering spores (mycotoxins) are much more serious than spores.

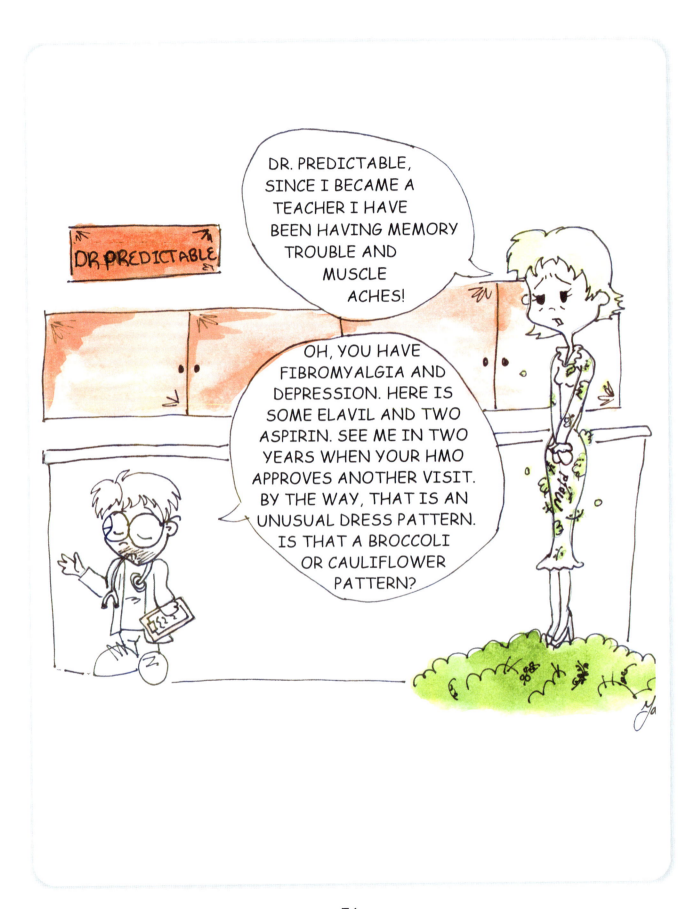

Vague Cloudy Medical Diagnoses for Mold Illness

Physicians see many patients each day with mold illness. Mold illness symptoms have been listed in earlier sections. But since physicians have no training in diagnosing mold toxins, they have to call it something. Some of the current diagnoses are: Fibromyalgia, Chronic Fatigue Syndrome, Depression, Somatization, Munchhausen Syndrome and Hypochondriasis.

For example, Fibromyalgia is a collection of symptoms that include widespread aches, pain, stiffness, tenderness, fatigue and sleep disturbance.

Chronic Fatigue Syndrome is also a collection of symptoms that include severe prolonged fatigue, memory deficits, reduced concentration, sore throat, tender lymph nodes, joint and muscle pain, headaches, poor sleep quality and poor recovery from exertion.

Depression can be a real biological illness. But often if you do not fit into routine medical diagnoses and you feel ill and sad, traditional physicians are left tagging you with the psychiatric diagnosis of depression.

Hypochondriasis is a label for those with significant anxiety. People with this psychiatric label have a wide range of physical symptoms and sensations magnified beyond their reality. These patients are felt to "doctor shop," annoy physicians and catastrophize their illness.

It is very helpful to our mold patients to perform mold testing of their exposure source, and to test their body using reliable and respected medical tests to show them results that prove the problem is "not in their head!"

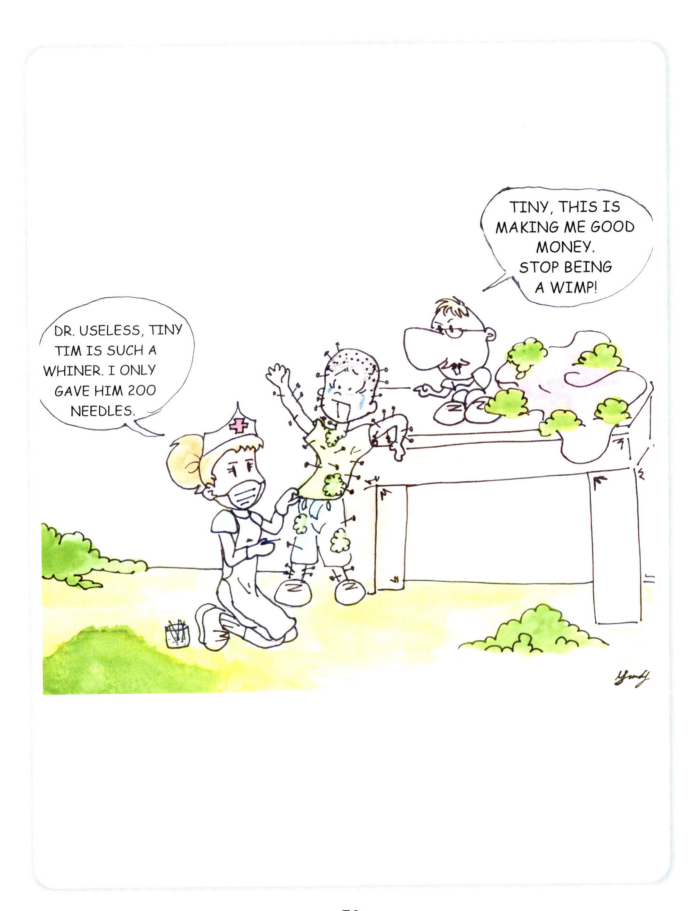

Allergy Trouble is NOT Mold Toxin Exposure

Indoor mold toxins cause hundreds of symptoms. A small number appear to be similar to routine allergies and include nasal symptoms, rashes and red eyes. Traditional medicine is interested in diagnosing special allergy antibody reactions and "selling" long-term prescriptions to soothe the symptoms. They diagnose the cause of this reaction or "allergy" by injecting a substance into the skin to see if they get a reaction.

While allergy testing has its place, it has nothing to do with a reaction to the biotoxin chemicals made by many different indoor molds.

Perhaps an analogy is comparing a person's reaction to ragweed pollen and their reaction to cyanide.

Allergists and physicians treating asthma offer a useful service, but as a trend their treatments do not help the effects of mold toxins. Also, in some cases, their use of steroids can lower crucial MSH that has twenty critical body roles. Of course if a person has asthma, they may need a steroid, since asthma is dangerous if not controlled.

In patients with mold toxicity, once they are removed from the mold source and treated for mold toxin exposure, some become free of these allergy-like symptoms and can stop taking their allergy medications.

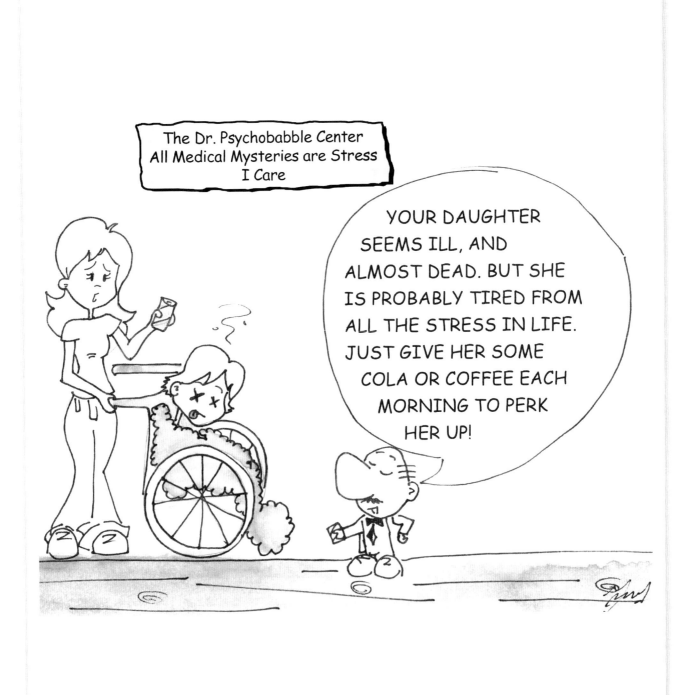

Indoor Mold: A Caring Physician is Not Enough

Some years ago, members of my family were dying of Lyme (another biotoxin illness), after dozens of physicians in five states were ineffective in treating them. So I found their treatment solutions myself.

Unfortunately, only a small number of physicians are self-trained to understand, diagnose and treat biotoxin illness.

Therefore, you will need to learn about this illness through self-study, since your sincere physicians may not be able to direct you. Indeed, you might have to buy them solid books on mold toxin illness for their library. Some will read them.

"MOLD!? I AM SURE THIS IS NOT A MOLD PROBLEM, BUT AN ALLERGY. MOLD MAKES CHEESE AND BEER AND IS PERFECTLY SAFE! HOWEVER, TIM MIGHT HAVE A LITTLE OLE' ALLERGY TO MOLD. IF HE DOES, I WILL JUST USE A TON OF ANTIHISTAMINES, ANTIBIOTICS AND STEROIDS. NO BIG DEAL. AND IF THAT DOES NOT HELP, WE CAN ALWAYS SPEND YEARS LOOKING INTO WHEAT AND DAIRY ALLERGIES, OR ALLERGIES TO HUNDREDS OF THINGS HE CAN AVOID ONE BY ONE ..."

DR. USELESS

A PROUD MEMBER OF TUMS

Alternative Medicine Does Not Get It Either

Some progressive physicians have come to the conclusion that traditional medicine has many blind spots. So they have added some extra training to their basic medical school education.

They offer some useful principles. For example, they feel that wheat gliadin protein can make some patients feel unhealthy, and so they suggest that diets should avoid wheat, corn syrup or dairy. This probably has merit in some mold patients, because their immune system can become much more reactive to some things like wheat gliadin protein.

Other progressive physicians also discuss the need for preventive treatments: taking high-quality nutrients, replacing low levels of natural hormones, removing excess heavy metals, and taking probiotics or the "good" bacteria required for healthy intestinal function.

Mold toxins are used in war and are very serious. Modifying your diet, taking nutrients or using natural hormones will not remove mold toxins.

Many traditional physicians do not accept alternative treatments. That is a shame, because these can make a patient with mold illness feel better. For example, some mold toxins make important hormones fall to useless levels. Supplementing with natural bio-identical hormones might help you feel better. This is not a cure, but it might help.

Unfortunately, many traditional physicians only get their education from a few conservative journals controlled by huge pharmaceutical corporation money. These physicians prescribe strong steroids and antibiotics, which usually are Band-Aids with little long-term effect on mold toxin illness.

Unfortunately, some of the most uncreative and useless forces in medicine are state medical boards, specialty societies and Ivy League centers, controlled by lawyers, corrupt "experts" and drug grants. They limit new clinical thinking and slow the use of practical clinical care solutions.

Mold Illness Hurts Relationships

The brain is the most sensitive organ, and small mycotoxin exposures can have big consequences.

Look over the list below. Do you see any of these front brain signs in your child, yourself or school staff? Are any of these changes new and associated with exposure to water damage and/or a moldy smelling home or school?

- Moody and irritable
- Rigidity
- Restlessness
- Poor insight
- New distractibility
- Trouble finishing a task
- Impulsivity: acting eccentrically with money, drinking, drugs, sex, unwanted pregnancy, or speech content
- Decreased speech speed and smoothness
- Decreased coordination
- Stress with transitions or change
- Routine lateness
- Limited empathy
- New immature silliness
- Social deficits – making other people uncomfortable
- Poor awareness of emotional or verbal boundaries

An Indoor Mold or Biotoxin Symptom Checklist

There is no single test that will show if you are ill from mold. But now some solid blood tests exist which help point to a mold diagnosis. These tests are not the common simplistic organ failure labs people get at yearly physicals. These tests are also not simply traditional allergy testing. Many of these lab tests are described in a book I co-authored, **Mold Warriors: Fighting America's Hidden Health Threat**. These tests are commonly covered by most insurance plans.

There are many tests to choose from, but since most readers are not physicians, there is no point describing them. Further, even if you have mold toxin labs performed, your doctor may not have the basic knowledge to understand them. If a doctor really wants to treat mold illness they should read a number of books on mold illness, or send you to someone who is treating biotoxic mold.

However, one test is as simple as comparing yourself to your healthy peers. Look over the list on the next page and see how many fit you or your loved ones exposed to toxic mold species in a home, school or workplace. Mark each one that fits. It does not have to be extreme to be positive.

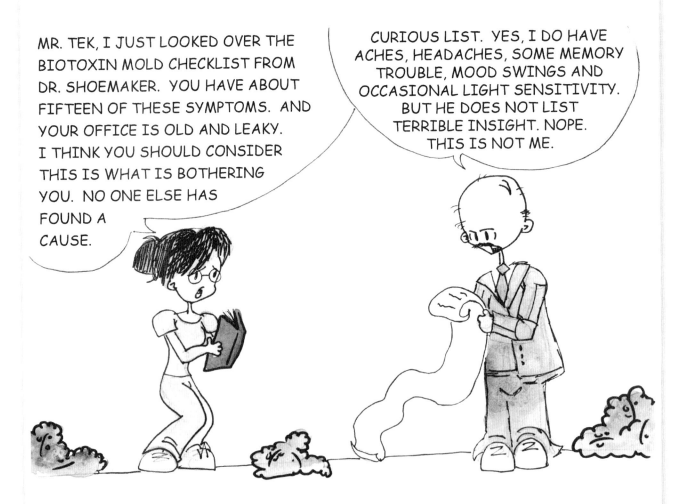

A Biotoxin Mold Checklist

Please look over these signs of mold and other biotoxins. If you fit seven of these you should consider a consult with a mold literate physician. Be honest and alert when filling out.

- Fatigue
- Weakness
- Aches
- Cramps
- Unusual Pain
- Ice Pick Pain
- Lightning Bolt Pain
- Headache
- Light Sensitivity
- Red Eyes
- Blurred Vision
- Tearing
- Sinus
- Cough
- Shortness of Breath
- Abdominal Pain
- Diarrhea
- Joint Pain
- Morning Stiffness
- Numbness
- Tingling
- Metallic Taste
- Vertigo
- Memory
- Confusion
- Poor Focus/Concentration
- Decreased Assimilation of New Knowledge
- Decreased Word Finding Ability
- Disorientation
- Skin Sensitivity
- Excessive Thirst
- Frequent Urination
- Static/Shocks
- Sweats - especially night sweats
- Mood Swings
- Temperature Regulation
- Appetite Swings

Most toxic mold exposed patients have an average of eighteen of these symptoms. However, some are really not in touch with their illness, and I would explore it further if just seven symptoms are present. For example, if you have lived or worked in a location with visible or musty mold, or have just seven of these, I would get the HLA and MSH labs and others in the following chapter.

(Source: Shoemaker, Schaller and Schmidt, *Mold Warriors: Fighting America's hidden health threat*. This can be ordered from www.moldwarriors.com or Amazon.com)

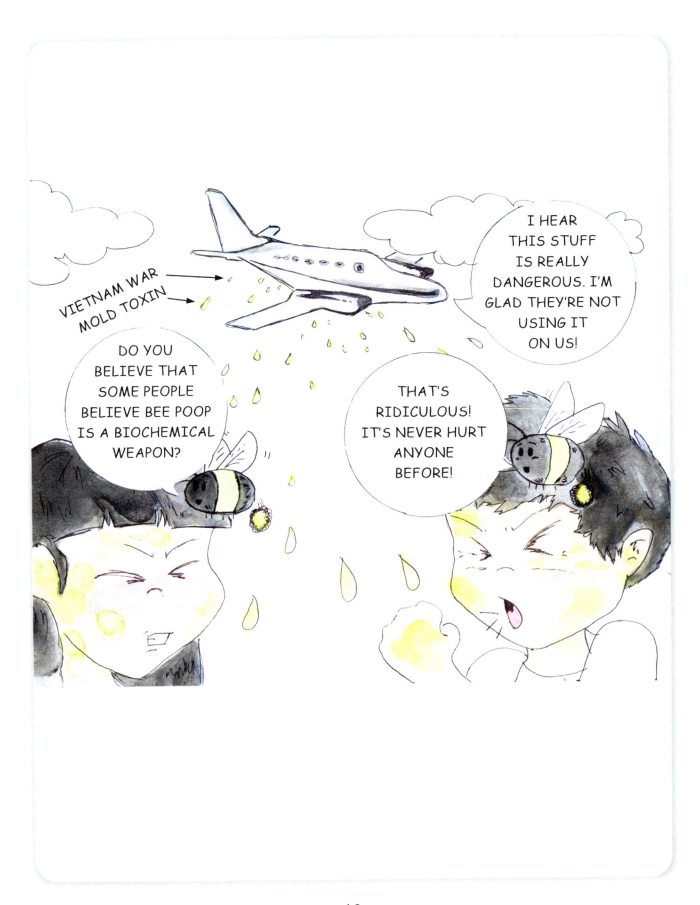

Mold Toxin Use in War: More Than a Runny Nose

According to research done by a military toxicologist, a respected Internist, the intelligence community, and the U.S. State Department, there is a strong belief mold toxins have been used in war. Mold toxins are very easy to make into weapons. One example is the clear mold biological warfare agents that caused deaths between 1975 and 1981 in Afghanistan, Laos and Kampuchea (Cambodia). Some of these agents included the mold toxin T-2 and were designed by the Soviet Union and its client states. Chemical and biological agents were delivered from aircraft spray tanks, helicopters, rockets, bombs, hand-held launchers and booby traps. T-2 is a common mold toxin present in water-damaged homes.

The air attacks in Laos were described as yellow rain, mist, smoke or yellow powder. Some attacks had other colored material. T-2 samples were collected from plastic and rocks surfaces, and were not found in areas that had not been attacked. Up to 32% of human samples were positive in mold warfare areas, and only 2% positive from non-attacked areas (perhaps from food with mold).

Bee Feces and Toxic Yellow Rain

Some scientists doubt weaponized mold toxins were the source of yellow rain, even though it is easy to make mold toxins by the ton, and the extracted mold toxins are usually yellow. They blame the yellow on the feces of vast swarms of bees that poop and clean themselves. Other researchers cannot understand how bee feces would make soldiers ill and die. While bees certainly do poop and clean, and some of it got into certain samples, the substance is not known to kill people.

Also, some samples with T-2 had polyethylene glycol, which is only found in manufactured materials, and is not found in nature.

Do Mold War Toxins Relate to You?

Testing of mold toxins on people is not usually performed. Low doses of war mold chemicals caused eye problems, tearing, blurred vision, skin symptoms, blisters, skin redness, rashes, burning, swelling, nausea, vomiting and intestinal discomfort. Canadian Medical forces found these types of symptoms in soldiers 100-300 meters from mold artillery devices exploded in former Cambodia. The symptoms took 2-5 minutes to start. (Many patients enter a moldy school, building, store or home and have many similar symptoms in a few minutes).

Others exposed to these war agents experienced nasal itching, pain, a runny nose, nosebleeds, a sore throat, coughing, shortness of breath, air hunger, chest pain, dizziness, headache, fatigue, a rapid heart, and voice changes. Perhaps you or your loved ones have experienced some of these symptoms.

Larger doses caused death in minutes to days after a "high dose" exposure. Some died of severe stomach bleeding and bleeding in the intestines.

Wannemacher RW Jr, Wiener SL. Trichothecene Mycotoxins. In: Zajtchuk R, Bellamy RF, eds. *Textbook of military medicine: Medical aspects of chemical and biologic warfare*. Washington, DC: Office of the Surgeon General at TMM Publications, Borden Institute, Walter Reed Army Medical Center; 1997:655-77.

Mold Toxins Given as Cancer Treatment

A common way to kill cancer is to give a person a modest poison and let the fast growing tumor take up the poison faster than other body cells and eventually die. In other words, fast growing cells like tumors die easier than other human cells with chemotherapy treatment.

Mold toxins are poisons and were examined for their ability to kill cancer.

Simply, it seems that there is really no such thing as a useful or safe dose of a mold toxin. Patients were given anguidine, a mold toxin, to try to kill their cancer. Instead, the tumors were not hurt and the patients had a wide range of side effects:

- Nausea
- Vomiting
- Diarrhea
- Burning red skin
- Confusion
- Trouble thinking
- Walking trouble
- Chills
- Fever
- Life threatening low blood pressure
- Hair loss

Goodwin W, Haas CD, et. al. Phase I evaluation of anguidine (diacetoxyscirpenol), NSC-141537). *Cancer*. 1978;4:23-26

Murphy WK, Burgress MA, et. al. Phase I clinical evaluation of anguidine. *Cancer Treat Rep*. 1978:62:1497-1502

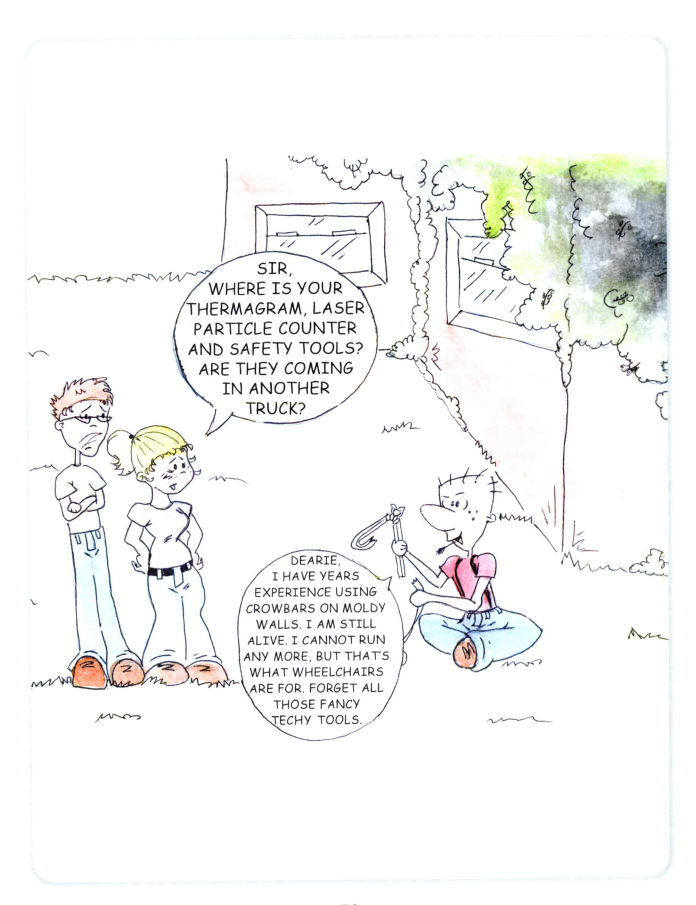

Need Good Remediation? Become Governor!

Most Governor's mansions are old. Like many old government buildings many of these structures have indoor toxic mold. However, these extensively remediated mansions mentioned below might be safer than your current home, and worth seeking the office of Governor. This option might be useful if you cannot afford a remediation of your current home or office.

- In 1995 the Texas Governor Mansion under Governor George W. Bush was remediated at a cost of $50,000.
- Louisiana Governor Kathleen Blanco left the Governor's mansion. The mansion is undergoing an $800K renovation, $500K of which is for mold removal.
- The South Carolina Governors Mansion was remediated for $5.6 million because of the black mold (stachybotrys) according to First Lady Jenny Sanford.
- North Carolina Governor Mike Easley moved his family out of the 114-year-old mansion because of an invasion by mold. It is growing under the wallpaper, around pipes and inside the heat and air ducts. The entire heat and air conditioning systems will be replaced for $3.5 million. The air systems are over 30 years old. This is the second time the mansion was remediated, since a million was spent five years ago for mold remediation. Since this is the second remediation, we suggest not running for the Governor of North Carolina until post-remediation testing proves the ancient structure is free of mold.

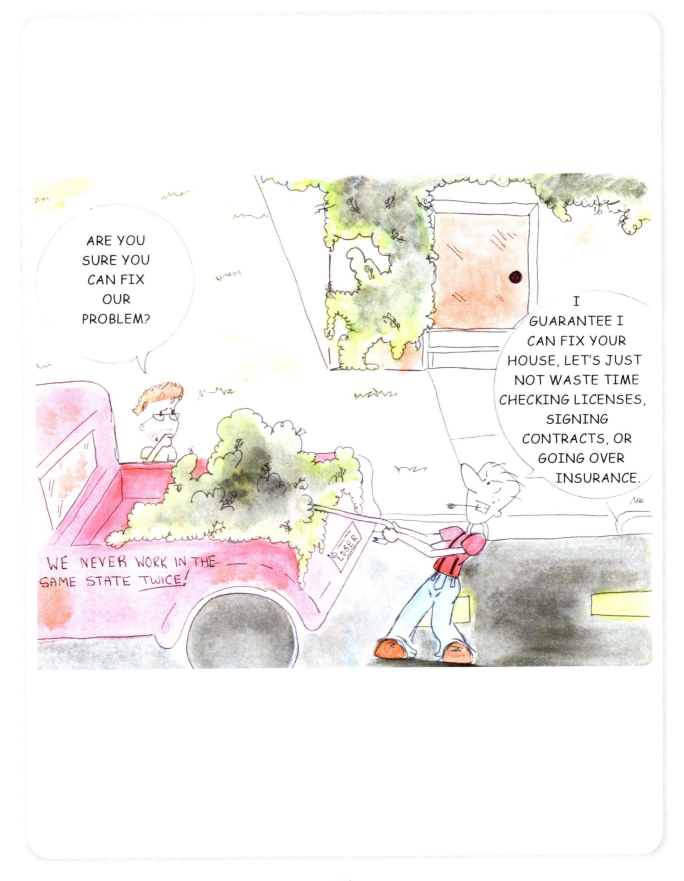

You Know You Have the Wrong Remediator When...

- He laughs when you ask if he has a contractor's license or a mold remediator certification or license.
- You ask if he has at least one million dollars in construction or mold insurance, and he falls on the ground convulsing with laughter. Take him out in a wheel barrel and dump the clown.
- He has no clue or concern about fixing the source of the moisture. He does not realize ignoring the source of the moisture problem will mean the mold will always come back.
- He has no plan to put up temporary walls with plastic wall sheeting to prevent mold dust and mold toxins from going all over your home.
- The remediator wears no protective mask or gloves.
- He has no plan to channel moldy dust from the work area outside through a window or external door.
- The remediator plans to carry unsealed material through your home.
- You ask him who will do the "post-remediation mold testing" he looks at you like you have ten heads.
- He does not use a HEPA vacuum to clean up after himself.
- He does not seal off your air conditioning ducts to prevent mold spores and dust from going all over your home during the remediation work.
- He is foggy from his past jobs. He does not know how to contain mold dust, since he is showing signs of mold exposure. So do not expect him to know how to prevent the release of moldy dust throughout your home.

Humidity Meters: A Cheap Way to Test the Waters

When I talk about checking out the humidity in your home or work, I am very serious about "testing the waters" or the water in the air. You may be stunned to find that some areas of your home or work are often over 65% humidity. Dust mites grow at 55% and mold grows when humidity is over 65%.

I routinely find humidity over 65% in various parts of homes.

- Bathrooms are notorious for high humidity and most do not have exhaust fans that run automatically until the humidity is low enough.
- Kitchens and family rooms often have high humidity from cooking, using the dishwasher and the humidity from people's bodies.
- Near the washing machine
- Basements, crawl spaces and attics
- Leaks from pipes, windows, roof joints and ice dams

Buying a Portable Small Humidity Meter

We suggest getting an electronic meter since they are more accurate than older mechanical devices. You can get one at Wal-Mart or Home Depot for under $25.00.

Keeping Humidity Healthy

1) Run your AC as much as is affordable since in the cooling process water condenses on the air handler coils and humidity is drained away.

2) To reduce moisture levels in the air, repair leaks, increase ventilation (if outside air is cold and dry), or dehumidify. Have any dehumidifier connected so its water run off goes outside the home.

3) Put a Humidistat on your AC control. These are very inexpensive and will allow your AC to keep the humidity low.

4) If you ever see any leaks, condensation or wet spots … eliminate the source and dry the moisture in 48 hours.

5) Make sure your AC unit is inspected every year. The drain can easily become clogged, and a 1/2 cup of bleach every four months might help keep it open. If it clogs, the air conditioning system's drip pan will overflow with water. This will result in mold at the bottom of your AC. This mold then gets sucked into your AC and spreads throughout the house.

6) Vent clothes dryers to the outdoors. Make sure the dryer hose is properly connected with no leaks.

7) During winter months your skin may become too dry due to low humidity. But you can still get mold growth in low humidity if moisture is condensing on cool or cold surfaces.

8) The ground around your home should have a slope that drains water away from the foundation.

9) Avoid storing organic materials such as paper, books, cardboard

boxes, clothes, etc., in humid locations (such as in non air-conditioned basements, crawl spaces or garages).

10) Use dehumidifiers in humid areas such as basements that read over 60% on your humidity meter.

11) If visitors mention a "musty smell" listen very closely, since your nose quickly becomes desensitized to a smell. Try to smell the odor after you have been away for some days, but listen to the reports of others.

12) Keep gutters clean and make sure down spouts carry the water several feet from the house.

13) While pollen levels and many allergy symptoms fall during a rain storm, mold grows in moisture. Windows and doors should be kept closed when it is damp and humid outside.

Training Your Eyes to Discern Indoor Mold in Sixty Seconds

Mold That is Obvious to Anyone Who is Sober

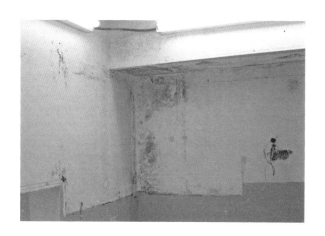
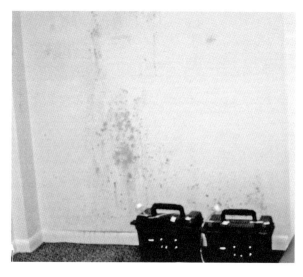
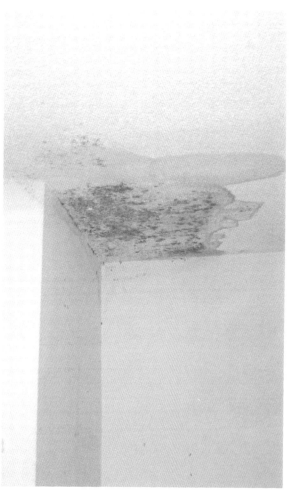

New Construction and New Mold

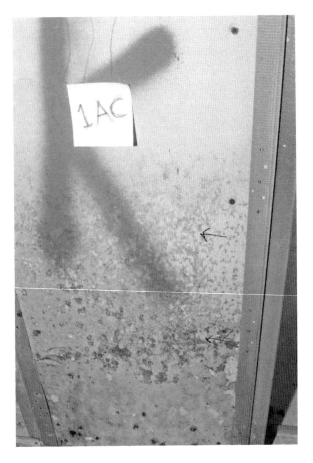

Moisture on metal can support mold in dusty construction sites.

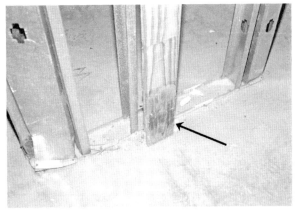

Wood is often left outside or in moist storage areas during construction. Then, it is often used in construction without removing the mold. (The mold is located on the bottom of this board).

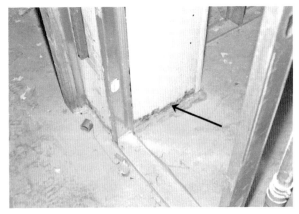

Here is clear mold located between the floor and a wall joint.

Important Mold Lessons From Pictures

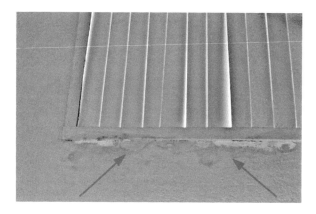

Windows are often poorly installed. Water can occasionally enter around them, as is seen in this window.

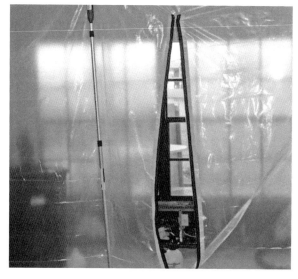

Any remediator who is not using some type of plastic wall, should be asked to leave. A remediator who does not set up a barrier is dangerous.

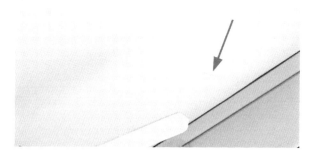

Many ceilings have clear evidence of water damage. Here a small crack shows a small water leak. Be suspicious of newly painted walls and ceilings hiding past or present leaks and mold.

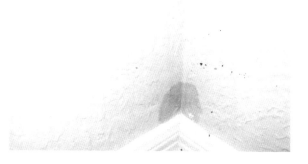

Building joints are places where water can easily collect from a leak. Some people paint over these stains just before they try and sell their home.

Important Mold Lessons From Pictures

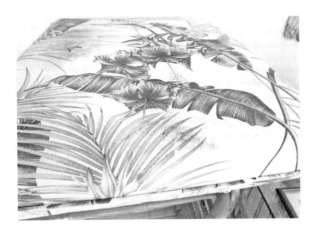

Furniture cloth exposed to excess humidity can develop mold. Most moldy fabrics should be discarded.

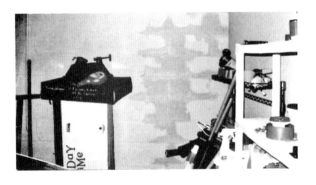

Water leaks are commonly treated casually. This type of leak can create significant mold on the wall and materials stored in the basement.

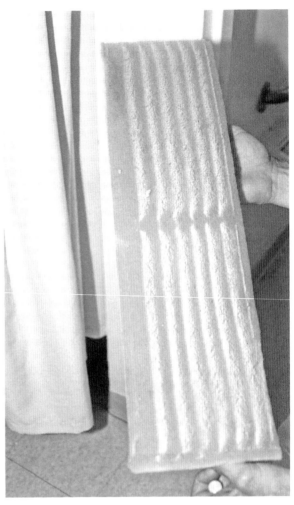

Here is one of many junk filters that do not filter well, and allow poor air flow with possible condensation. They allow dust, which is mold food, to eventually fill the air ducts

Surprises Behind Pretty Paint, Wallboard and Wallpaper

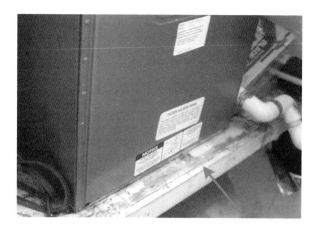

Air Handlers should be inspected regularly to make sure dust is cleaned off the inside cooling coils (inside the silver air handler) and the drainage tube is draining away water. Here we see mold on the wood base of an air handler, most likely from a drainage pan overflow.

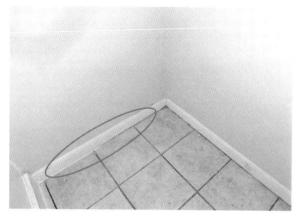

Unless you look carefully, you might think this baseboard merely has a little dust on the edges. But look at what is behind the walls in the "after" picture below.

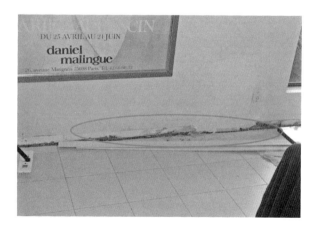

Removing baseboards is often a very good way to check for mold in the walls.

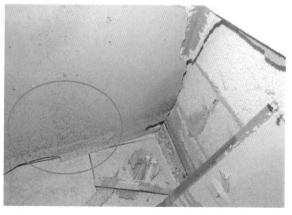

After the wall and baseboard materials are removed, the mold is obvious.

Surprises Behind Pretty Paint, Wallboard and Wallpaper

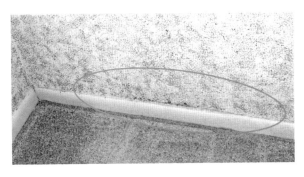

Notice the mold peaking out at the bottom of the wallpaper. Plenty of mold is under the carpet and behind the wallpaper.

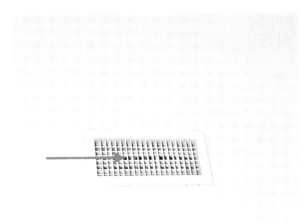

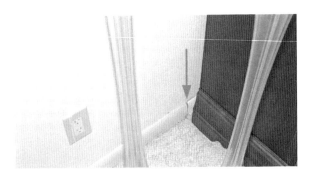

Brownish mold is at the top of the baseboard just behind the wood furniture.

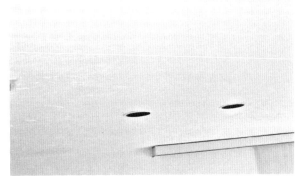

If air ducts are not clean they will grow mold on the dust in the ducts. Also, they carry mold from moldy rooms to the rest of your home, workplace and school.

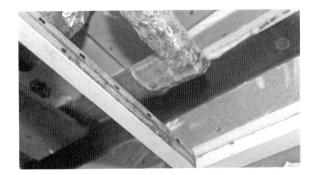

Note the rusty metal which is in the false ceiling metal framing. Rust means water, and water means mold. Mold just loves wet ceiling tiles.

Powerful Lessons from Finland

Dr. Meklin studied thirty-two Finnish school buildings, and over 5,000 students. She discovered that:

1. Finland schools were not properly ventilated in order to save on energy costs. Poor ventilation contributes to moisture damage by increasing water condensation.
2. When a school's moisture damage and mold problems were fixed, kids returned to good health.
3. Schools with good ventilation and no moisture damage had very low instances of diseases related to indoor air quality.
4. School air pollution included bacteria, viruses, and toxic substances from deteriorating furnishings, carpets, and cleaning materials.
5. The highest disease-producing molds in Finnish schools were Penicillium and Aspergillus.

Sample symptoms reported by Finnish school children in mold-contaminated schools included:

- Fatigue
- A 350% higher rate of asthma
- Respiratory infections
- Eye irritation
- Increased visits to physicians and use of antibiotics

Symptoms Finnish school personnel reported:

- Fatigue
- Headache
- Stuffy nose
- Eye irritation
- Nausea
- Sleeping difficulties

Again, this is yet another study – and there are too many with similar results to include them all – in which we see that categorizing mold toxin illness as merely a case of a runny nose and a little asthma is simply to deny quality scientific and medical evidence.

Laboratory Testing for Mold Symptoms

Go Beyond Simple Allergy Labs With a Small Sample of Special Mold Labs

Many physicians and patients think that mold merely affects your nasal areas and lungs. So they think a "full laboratory" evaluation is simply allergy testing and perhaps some special breathing tests called "Pulmonary Function Tests." While these have a use, they are limited tests and miss the point that mold toxins are always active throughout the entire human body, possibly hurting any body organ or any chemical system.

Below we review select and special lab tests that are used to check for mold toxin symptoms. Your family doctor could order these tests if you are concerned about mold exposure. Although very important, these tests are not commonly done. They should be.

We are not trying to turn you into "little doctors," and so we will try to avoid medical jargon. But some of these lab tests and explanations can be a little technical. What matters most is that you get the test. After that, you can explore any abnormal result.

Children usually prefer getting as little blood work as possible. The use of a compounded pain relieving cream or prescription EMLA numbing cream can reduce pain if applied an hour before blood testing. The cream should be applied to the inner elbow joints generously, and kitchen plastic wrap should hold the cream tightly on the skin. We also routinely use 0.5 mg of Xanax to calm frightened children. They are very thankful.

In a perfect world, we would suggest large adolescents and adults get as many of the lab tests as possible. Below we discuss several of the most important ones for children.

Melanocyte Stimulating Hormone (MSH)

Perhaps one of the most serious blind spots in current medical practice is an ignorance of the massive role that MSH plays in the body. It is a major controlling hormone involved in up to twenty functions. If it is low you could have any one of thirty different problems. It is not an optional lab test, and I (Schaller) feel it should be part of an average medical workup in all Americans. The most common cause of a very low MSH in my patients is exposure to biotoxins. If it is below 35 according to LabCorp ranges, it is low. And many youth with biotoxin exposure can have less than 20. In addition to mold toxins, Lyme biotoxins and severe inflammation also can reduce MSH levels.

You might recall from high school biology that MSH is involved in skin color. Now we know it has many other serious health roles in the body. In fact, pharmaceutical companies around the world are seeing the many roles for this hormone and are scrambling to make it in a slightly altered form so they can patent it. They expect to make a fortune.

So what do all these drug companies know? What role does MSH have besides tanning and skin color?

MSH's Massive Role in the Body

MSH has many roles, but a low MSH does not mean a child will have all the problems listed below.

Memory and learning: If your child has a low MSH, then they will have a harder time recalling classwork. A child with a low MSH may seem forgetful and may struggle to stay on top of school work.

I wonder, how many children across America receive special education because of a reduced MSH? Since this is not routine medicine, we do not know yet. But it appears quite common in our patients with mold toxin poisoning or tick-borne Lyme disease.

Attention will fall in children or adults as MSH drops. I have repeatedly had patients called "ADHD" or "ADD," but these symptoms often started after they were ten years old. ADHD and ADD do not suddenly start in adolescence!

Obesity (or too thin): Typically, children and adults with a low MSH gain weight. Often they gain a significant amount of weight. Perhaps some people try to feel better by eating. But others gain weight with only moderate eating. Commonly, people with low MSH see their weight drift higher and higher. Diets may help somewhat, but people do not get the results they expect from their diet. They lose five pounds instead of fifteen. A small minority struggle to maintain their body fat, and start to look waif-like. Some of these exercise massive amounts to create natural opioids to feel better.

Pain relief: MSH encourages production of your natural opioids. If your MSH is low, you will feel aches and pains more often. Some youth complain of headaches. Others report joint pain, which is often called "growth pains." Further, you may be more inclined to do addictive, impulsive or pleasurable behaviors, in an effort to feel "normal" or "right" again. These addictive behaviors are very diverse. Low MSH promotes alcoholism, illegal drug use, binge eating, sexual experimentation, impulsive exercise, intense work, speed driving, thrill seeking actions, pornography addiction, and rage. With binge work, a person does not want to stop working because once they stop, they do not feel "right." Impulsive activity also may create a small amount of natural pain killing chemicals. And patients with rage may feel briefly "better" after a "blowup" for a similar reason.

Flat or bored mood: Having an MSH deficiency can reduce your feeling of joy. A person can be left with a malaise that is often different than typical depression.

Increased inflammation: MSH has strong affects on inflammation chemicals. If MSH drops, it will allow inflammation chemicals to increase. Inflammation causes increased pain, a depressed or irritable mood, increased agitation and increased blood clots that may increase heart attacks and strokes. Low MSH is also associated with an increase in lung inflammation or asthma, in addition to inflamed intestinal disorders.

Decreased coping ability: Low MSH makes it hard for body organs and the brain to handle personal stress.

Energy changes: In our experience, some patients with low MSH have increased fatigue and are listless. Some patients have both agitation and fatigue simultaneously.

Nerve repair: Throughout his or her life, the average person suffers many injuries that can hurt neurons – falls, car accidents, sports accidents, and simple aging. In addition to these, it appears low MSH may slow nerve repair.

Low libido or erection problems: Both genders have a significant drop in free testosterone in their 40's. For some it is over a 50% drop. This can make sex as interesting as a sewer. Men with a low MSH can also find that their genital plumbing is not functioning, not merely because of low testosterone or very low estrogen, which can cause a low libido, but because they have abnormally low MSH. For libido, women need a little testosterone, estrogen and progesterone. But if MSH is low, these hormones usually are also impaired, and libido can be affected. While a low libido might be good for adolescents, it is not a "benefit" one can pick with a low MSH – you get other negatives.

Excessive urination or mouth dryness: While this is often seen as a sign of diabetes, few physicians realize a low MSH can also cause this annoying symptom. Children dislike having to go to the bathroom more than their friends. They feel they look peculiar. Also, this unique form of urination removes salt from the body. Others have uncomfortably dry mouths that do not respond well to treatment.

Body temperature: Some children or adults have flashes of hot or cold sensations.

Testing MSH

Please do not go to just any laboratory. LabCorp offers the most meaningful clinical results. If you want a doctor to order a test for you, you will need to have all the material in this chapter in hand. And you will particularly need the material below, which lists the test code and the name of the special kits needed. LabCorp patient locations for a useful MSH can be found on the Internet at: www.LabCorp.com.

Please make sure the lab has a special test kit in stock before you go – the Trasylol kit.

Most physicians would not have the training to do this test in their office. So if an office clerk says they can, I would ask if they have any "Trasylol kits" in stock to be sent to LabCorp. After this blows them away, perhaps they might realize they are not equipped and will send you to a local LabCorp center.

Does MSH Replacement Exist?

Currently, the use of bio-identical MSH is not FDA approved. While a form exists that is a human, rat and mouse form – it is the same in all three mammals – it is not available for clinical use. Amazingly, it seems the NIH is not doing studies on this major hormone. Yet, many drug companies are scrambling to get patents. China is making this in many different factories. And an Australian pharmaceutical company has invented a patch delivery form. Hopefully, some drug company will have this approved in the USA soon, and patients with MSH deficiency will be able to use a patch or transdermal cream to replace their low MSH. Of course, many patients have their MSH return to normal after using Cholestyramine, which is a prescription mold toxin binding medication, and staying out of moldy homes or schools. (We will discuss cholestyramine in the binders section later).

Leptin and Obesity

Leptin is made by fat cells and is supposed to stop fat production and reduce appetite. Many things can mess up this function. For example, leptin function is often affected by biotoxins. Mold biotoxins ultimately cause leptin resistance, meaning that leptin does not turn on its receptor. As a result, the body makes much more than it needs and your blood levels shoot up. So leptin levels commonly become abnormal in a person who cannot remove mold toxins. These individuals become bloated and puffy and have trouble losing weight. They might lose some weight with great effort, but not as much as they should.

Sick Building Syndrome often causes blood leptin to go far above the normal range. If you or your child are no longer exposed to mold toxins, the leptin level might go down on its own. Yet for some patients, they will need to remove the mold toxins in their body by using a binding agent to normalize leptin. The most commonly used medication for this purpose is cholestyramine, which uniquely binds a vast number of mold toxins and other biological toxins in the intestines. The mold toxins are then passed out of the body in your stool. So taking Cholestyramine at one to two doses/day for children and four doses/day for adults after the mold exposure is gone can lower leptin levels. Furthermore, you can measure leptin levels to track your improvement – it should fall as you remove mold toxins from your body and avoid moldy schools and homes. If it does not return to normal, consider a consultation with a physician who specializes in mold toxin removal. You can get this test at any lab and one possible diagnostic code is 253.2.

Mold with Lyme Disease or Other Infections Routinely Missed

The number one vector illness in the U.S. is Lyme disease. It is found in every state and is rarely reported to state agencies. Indeed, one study showed that only one in 40 positive Lyme patients were reported to the state and the CDC. Lyme is carried by ticks that are often no bigger than a poppy seed and are rarely visible (unlike the large ticks found on dogs). Tiny deer tick nymphs sit in 2 inch grass and carry 100,000 Lyme spirochetes. They inject a painkiller, an antihistamine and anti-clotting chemicals to make their bite invisible.

We have found that some patients have both mold toxin illness and Lyme disease. Typically, this condition is missed because of the use of improper or inadequate laboratory testing.

If you want to rule out Lyme, consider using IGeneX labs, which is a Medicare CLIA-approved lab with exceptional blind negative and blind positive results. They do not use a single Lyme test strain from Europe or a single state. They also do not exclude key search proteins because of legal patents. Rather, they grow out and harvest the Lyme so that they offer equal and complete amounts of Lyme proteins. The tests use these proteins to bind to your antibodies. Furthermore, IGeneX's blind testing is far better than the published results of many labs. So, if you are relying on a lab that doesn't use proteins specific for Lyme strains found throughout the USA, good luck!

We have seen individuals who had vivid bull's-eye rashes from Northern states come back fully negative after 1-5 months. They had clear symptoms that were not treated due to common junk labs coming back "negative." They were positive with IGeneX testing. Why stress this material? Some people have been exposed to mold and also pick up a tiny poppy-seed-sized deer tick along the way. So, they have mold illness and Lyme. You can order a test kit and mailer from IGeneX at 800-832-3200. Your physician will have to fill out an order sheet for you once you receive the kit.

Dr. Schaller is writing a pediatric tick-borne infection book with a Connecticut pediatrician who has treated 9,000 children with Lyme and other tick infections. In the meantime, for more information, log onto Dr. Schaller's web site, www.personalconsult.com, for over 140 Lyme disease articles.

VIP – A Powerful New Body Substance Routinely Ignored

Vasoactive Intestinal Polypeptide (VIP) is a very strong chemical in our bodies that dampens inflammation and immune reactivity. For years prednisone and other steroids have been the main treatment for most severe inflammatory disorders. But they have many problems with their long-term use, so we are exploring alternative treatments. VIP works throughout the body on many cells and inflammation locations to reduce a wide range of inflammation illnesses in animals, such as stopping multiple-sclerosis-like damage, reducing cell death, rheumatoid arthritis, Crohn's disease, septic shock and transplant rejection. VIP may soon have a role in treating patients with autoimmunity, excess immune reactivity, excess inflammation problems and organ transplants. (Some of these benefits may come from decreasing granzyme, perforin and FasL).

The test can be performed by LabCorp and requires the special chilled trasylol tube used in MSH tests. The lab code is 010397 with possible diagnostic codes of 787.91, 259.9 and 780.8.

A Small Sample of VIP References for Your Physician

Amazingly, there are over 10,000 references to VIP or Vasoactive intestinal peptide among PubMed's 11 million medical references, but many physicians have not been trained in its importance. Many companies are designing anti-inflammation medications using VIP, and until one is FDA approved, this hormone might be ignored. However, if you or your physician want an introduction to VIP all they have to do enter the words: "Vasoactive intestinal peptide." when visiting the web site http://www.ncbi.nlm.nih.gov/entrez/query.fcgi.

Below we have listed four references to help ignite the interest of your physician, any other health care provider, or yourself.

Abad C, Gomariz RP, Waschek JA. Neuropeptide Mimetics and Antagonists in the Treatment of Inflammatory Disease: Focus on VIP and PACAP. *Curr Top Med Chem*. 2006;6:151-63.

Yasmina Juarranz, Catalina Abad, Carmen Martinez, Alicia Arranz, Irene Gutierrez-Canas, Florencia Rosignoli, Rosa P Gomariz, Javier Leceta. Protective effect of vasoactive intestinal peptide on bone destruction in the collagen-induced arthritis model of rheumatoid arthritis. *Arthritis Research & Therapy* 2005, 7:R1034-R1045.

Fernandez-Martin A, Gonzalez-Rey E, Chorny A, Ganea D, Delgado M. Vasoactive intestinal peptide induces regulatory T cells during experimental autoimmune encephalomyelitis. *Eur J Immunol*. 2006;36:318-326.

Gonzalez-Rey E, Chorny A, Fernandez-Martin A, Ganea D, Delgado M. Vasoactive intestinal peptide generates human tolerogenic dendritic cells that induce CD4 and CD8 regulatory T cells. *Blood*. 2006;107:3632-3638.

The Miracle of Thermal Cameras – Why Every "Mold Expert" Must Use Them

Thermography is often used to find problems with electrical systems by looking for hot spots. Unfortunately, this common practice of top electricians has not become the norm in evaluating water damage.

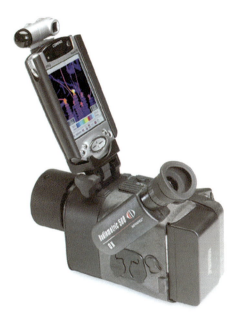

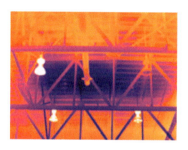

The dark blue color is a sign of moisture in the roof. After taking this image, Dr. Rosen promptly found that the roofing was wet and leaking in this exact dark blue spot.

This is a very special tool in mold detection – a thermographic camera. It allows a modern mold investigator and remediator to locate the source and extent of moisture that causes the mold growth.

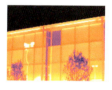

The blue window in the upper middle of this store front has a thermal image with an energy leak.

Color thermographic cameras start at $10,000. So only those very serious and striving for high professionalism have them.

Every day thousands of homes and other buildings undergo extensive renovation. Many of these structures have moisture and mold damage. I wonder how many construction renovators or remodeling builders have a thermographic camera? Or are they working in the dark?

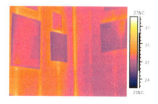

Thermal image of a wall with drywall over vertical solid wood joints. The air between the wood framing is hot and shows up various shades of pink-red.

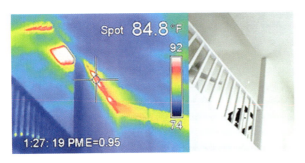

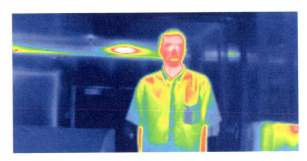

The left picture is an infrared image of the same ceiling area you see in the right photo. The blue color is in the mid 70's. The yellow, red and white colors are warmer, showing a defect in the roof in this home. By going up on the roof with a hose, we were able to show this hole leaked water which created extensive mold growth in the attic.

Thermal image of a man

The red color proves that humans are "hot heads" and lose a great deal of heat from their heads.

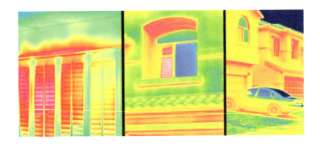

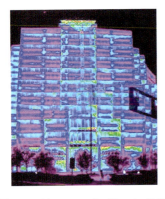

Thermal image of office building.

This huge glass covered building is pictured with a thermal camera which shows the indoor temperatures. Specifically, the blues and purples represent cool temperatures from the indoor AC. The green is from heat generated by ceiling lights. A thermal image of a large building can sometimes locate a water intrusion source in minutes.

Three thermal images of a housing development

Red equals the heat from the sun's rays, and is exhibited in red colors on the hot window shades (left image) and the garage doors (center and right image). Blue in this particular thermal machine means a cool temperature, such as from a home or car AC unit. The center window shows a cool window in blue from the cool air conditioned air. The right picture shows a car with the AC on high. In this same image a moist lawn with evaporating water cools the grass and creates a greenish color. Water on any surface can reduce the temperature of the object – just like human sweat cools the body. This feature of the thermal camera helps locate moisture pockets hidden from view.

Laser Particle Counters—Required for a Professional Remediation

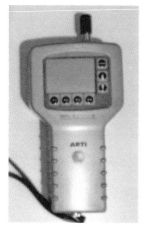

A Laser Particle Counter

The laser particle counter allows you to determine immediately where elevated levels of mold spores are located and if the mold remediation containment, e.g., a plastic barrier, is leaking and spreading mold spores throughout the house. If a piece of drywall is removed and mold spores are released, it can show immediately that the release is occurring. Anyone working in renovation should also have one, but this is almost never done. So builders removing old cabinets and old drywall routinely release indoor mold spores and toxic dust.

Why does a laser particle counter matter in the real world?

It is common for "Bubba" to try to clean up your mold or even to renovate with no concern for mold. If you want to know if they messed up and are contaminating the home or other building immediately, this machine will show mold particles of 5-10 micron increased 5 to 1000 fold. When these 5-10 micron size levels increase but the smaller sizes do not, you generally would assume mold spores.

Air sampling sent to a lab for analysis has a 2-3 day delay, but will let you know for sure these larger particles are mold spores.

A Real World Laser Particle Success Story

An elderly woman was very ill. Her doctor said her symptoms were most likely from mold. So she then had 3 different mold investigators come and take air samples. Each time it cost her $695 to $895. And each time the assessor said they could not find a problem. What was going on?

These sincere investigators were trying to hammer with a tooth pick. They did not have a laser particle counter. Her home had 30 year old carpets, and very old ratty stuffed sofas, from before the invention of the wheel. In rooms with such old rugs and furniture you will have some mold and some dust. And the modest levels of mold spores and heavy dust will be evenly dispersed everywhere in all the rooms from years of AC fan use, non-HEPA vacuums and human movement.

But the laser particle counter can handle old structures easily. Instead of taking a spore sample of the air filling an entire large room, you can test an exact spot. You can test for excess spores by a crack in the wall, or a suspicious light switch or a warped baseboard. Indeed, you can tap a wall and see if the 5-10 micron spores jump up in number. Dust has many sizes. But spores are generally in the 5-10 micron range.

So this elderly woman's son brought in a mold remediator with a laser particle counter. The investigator with the particle counter found the problem in about 10 minutes. The roof around the chimney was leaking and mold was growing in the adjacent wall. Easy to fix. Three weeks later the elderly lady was feeling much better.

Blind Insurance Companies

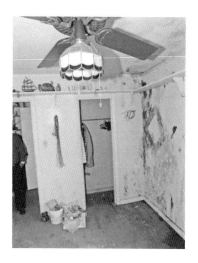

Left – A hurricane's high winds caused this roof leak and mold. The insurance company states that they cannot be sure that the water damage was actually a result of roof damage. The homeowner is an attorney, which is a useful training to have when fighting to have an insurance company acknowledge the obvious.

Water-Soaked Walls: Some Basics to Save You

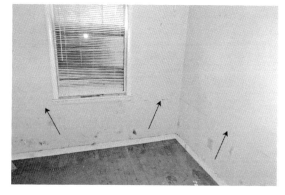

Right – In this image you can see a line two feet up from the floor. It is a water line from a flood. Millions of homes have had floods, hurricanes or severe water leaking. If the water has been in a structure for three days, one should assume massive mold damage. In this image, for example, it is common for all the walls to be filled with mold. Why? Because water at this volume will soak into the walls. Once the water on the floor is dried up, water or high humidity typically remains inside the wall cavity for days or weeks resulting in hidden mold.

A thermogram should also be used after a flood if any electrical device is in use, since it often shows areas of excess heat and electrical damage. We suggest that a licensed electrician confirm that electrical wiring is safe in any home which has had water fill a wall.

What is a Healthy Humidity Level?

Humidity should be at least 40%. If it is less than 40% your skin and mucous membranes in your throat and nasal passages can crack. Humidity over 55% can allow for slight dust mite growth. Mold growth can start at humidity levels over 65%.

Humidity range 45-55% is ideal.

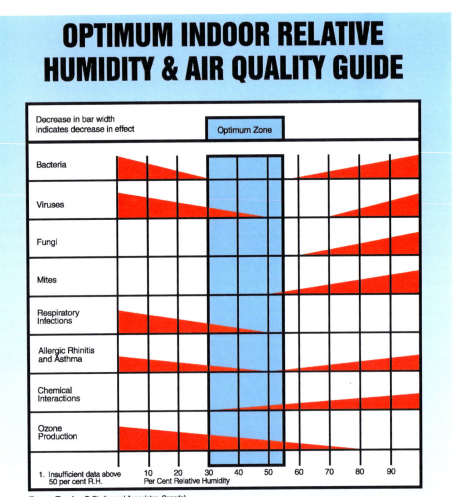

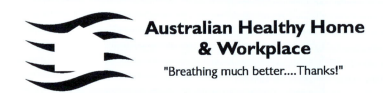

MERV 11 Filters

We regularly suggest that people have MERV 11 filters in their home and workplace. But some struggle to locate or understand the "MERV 11" rating. So below are a few different MERV 11 filters, and the print that can hide the MERV rating box. We have enlarged the MERV 11 marking for easy identification in the future.

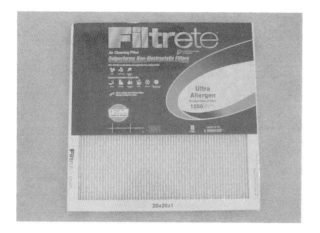
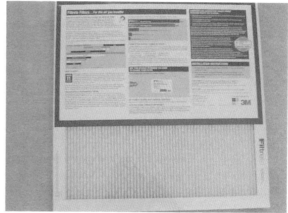

A 20 x 20 inch quality Filtrete MERV 11 filter (front and back). The front of the filter (above left) has many markings, but nothing about its MERV ability. The back panel (above right) has more scientific text and graphs than a PhD science course. See the MERV box on the back?

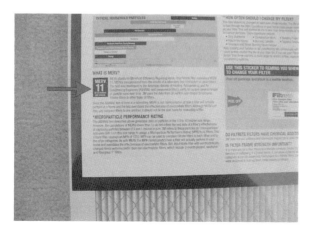

The MERV 11 rating box is on the bottom left of the back packaging materials in purple.

A scanned image of the same back showing how it is easy to miss the MERV 11 designation, because of the immense data on the back cover.

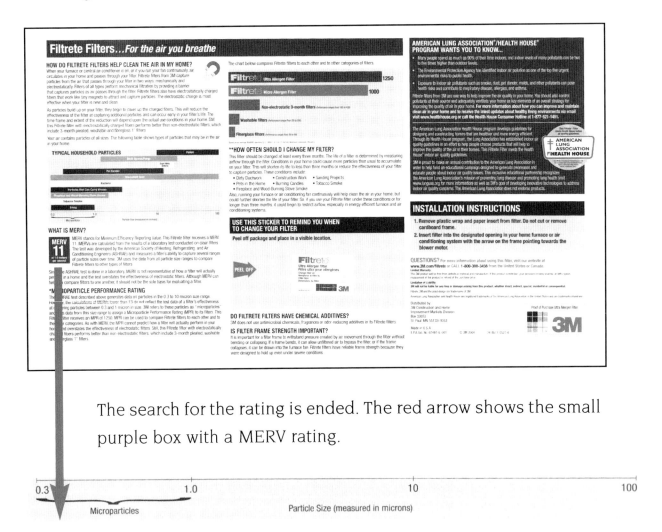

The search for the rating is ended. The red arrow shows the small purple box with a MERV rating.

WHAT IS MERV?

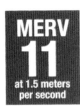

MERV stands for Minimum Efficiency Reporting Value. This Filtrete filter receives a MERV 11. MERVs are calculated from the results of a laboratory test conducted on clean filters. The test was developed by the American Society of Heating, Refrigerating, and Air Conditioning Engineers (ASHRAE) and measures a filter's ability to capture several ranges of particle sizes over time. 3M uses the data from all particle size ranges to compare Filtrete filters to other types of filters.

Since the ASHRAE test is done in a laboratory, MERV is not representative of how a filter will actually perform in a home and the test overstates the effectiveness of electrostatic filters. Although MERV can help you compare filters to one another, it should not be the sole basis for evaluating a filter.

Below is another filter with a different MERV rating placement. This MERV 11 rating is in the center of the back plastic covering. No rating is on the filter itself. Keep the bifocals handy if you intend to see the rating box.

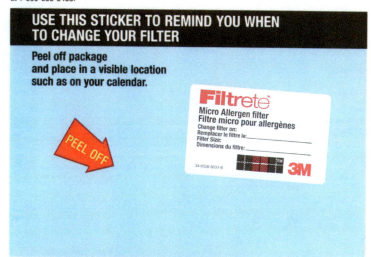

Finally, a third MERV placement is in a black box. In this filter the rating is found in the front upper right corner highlighted with an arrow.

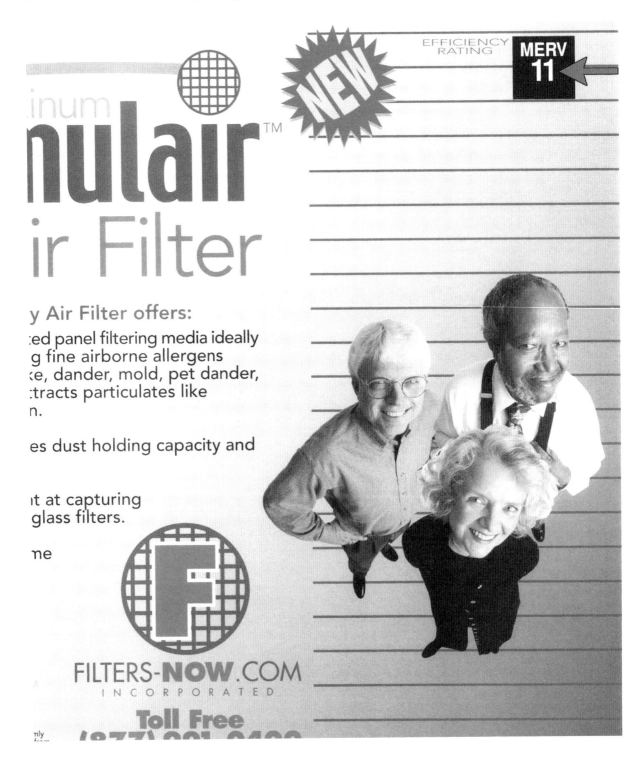

The Rosen $25.00 HEPA "Machine"

If you have a low mold problem and have done as much as you can to drop the indoor mold count, you can drop it even further with these types of mold dust removers. In some schools, we have found a clear spore count drop using these fans. While they do not replace sealing water leaks and removing indoor mold, they may help remove final low residues.

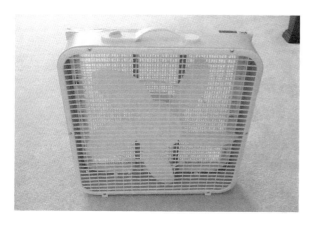

Start with a 20 inch box fan. They are available for $10-15.00.

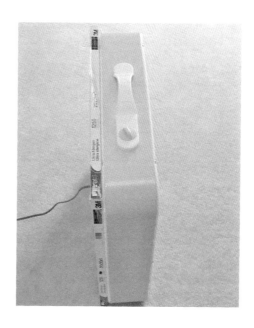

Side view of a MERV 11 filter attached to the back of the box fan. Place the filter with the small arrow on the top pointing forward, or in the direction of air flow. Attach the filter to the box fan with clear tape. If by accident you place the filter in the front of the box fan, the air will blow out the sides. The filter must be a 20 inch by 20 inch filter to fit the 20 inch box fan.

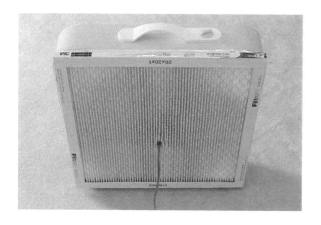

A neighbor accidentally purchased a box fan with the power cord coming out the center. A tiny cut and some tape fixed the problem, but buy one with the cord coming out the bottom or the top. This filter was used for three weeks, 24 hours a day on high, and it already shows some dust collection.

Air Handler Filter Slots

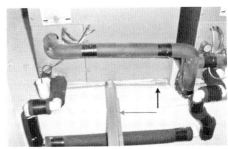

The silver metal strip in the photo (right, indicated by the red arrow) is the bottom cover for the thin space where a MERV 11 can sit. It is resting on the black foam-coated drainage tube. The black arrow shows the white and blue MERV 11 filter peeking out of the slot. After a filter is placed carefully into the bottom slot, this silver 1 inch plate would be replaced for a snug seal (noted by a circle).

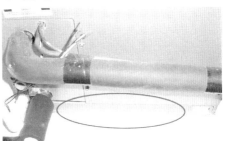

Here we see the silver filter plate in place. The red oval shows it is seated correctly at the bottom of the air handler. The black and white tubing coming out of the bottom of the air handler is the drainage tube that takes water away from the air handler. The water is collected when the warm inside air hits the cold coils. Adding bleach to the drain tube twice a year will help keep dirt, algae, and other junk from clogging these tubes. If they get blocked up, and you do not have a back up alarm, you can have water spill out and produce mold.

This air handler was DESIGNED so the drainage tube blocked the ability to place a filter in the air handler slit in the bottom. This is a clear construction defect. After some repeated firm appeals to the builder and the AC installation company, this was fixed. Filters can now be installed.

The best place to buy odd-shaped filters is at www.filters-now.com. Their toll-free phone and fax numbers are:
Ph: (877) 991-0400   Fax: (888) 823-6475

They can also talk to you about how to measure to get the correct size.

Portable HEPA Machines

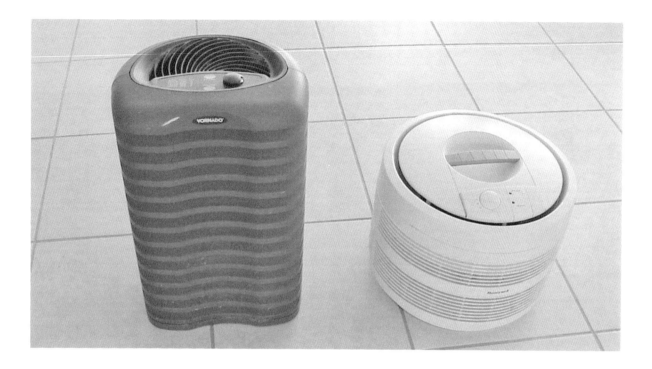

Portable air filters are generally overrated. First, if mold is in a home or building, the portable air filters will not successfully remove the billions of mold spores and toxin-filled dust. The "treatment" is not more portable air filters, but the removal of any water sources and the removal of the mold. Simply, you will never stop a gasoline fire until you shut off the gasoline valve.

Further, portable filter devices are very expensive. In one facility, a number of employees were ill from the moldy ceiling tiles. Their "solution" was to buy more and more filters. Friends were encouraged to join the "filter cult" to fight back the mold.

Eventually, the building leaks were fixed, and the employees did not need all their air filters. In retrospect, the portable filters only helped for a few weeks while the filters were new. They clogged rapidly with large and small dust particles and quickly lost their ability to filter.

Comparing Filters in Common Air Filtering Devices

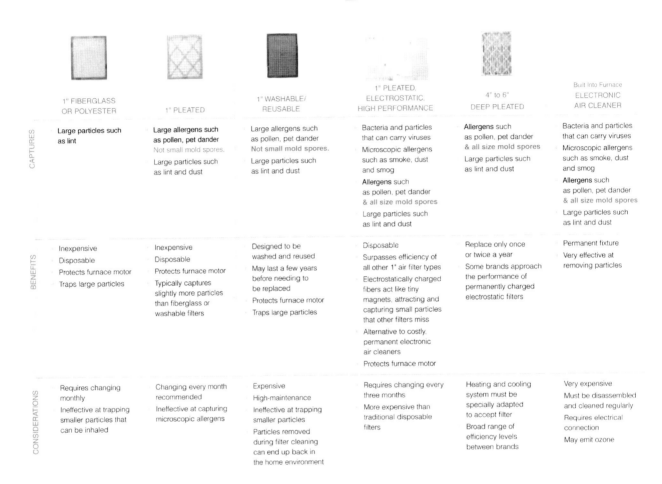

(Source: 3M Corporation's web site with some colored text inserts by Dr. Gary Rosen)

How To Change An Air Filter Without Filling Your Home With Mold Toxins

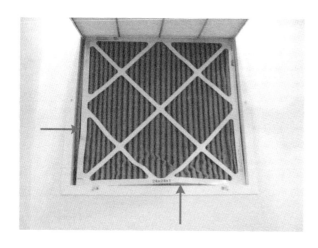

First, notice that the filter is not seated fully in the holder. Dirty air can pass unfiltered into the AC systems. And mold toxins that might have previously been collected on the surface of the filter could be pulled into the AC system. This was a white filter seven weeks ago. Better to have this junk in the disposable filter and not in your body or on your furniture.

Time to change the filter, but let's do so smartly.

To prevent the mold dust and spores from falling all over your home, turn off the AC fan and place a bag right under the filter before you remove it.

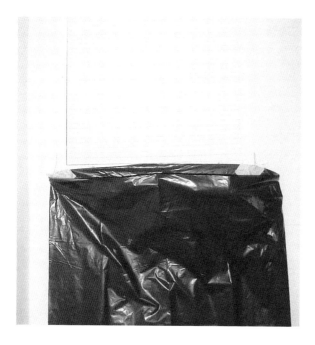

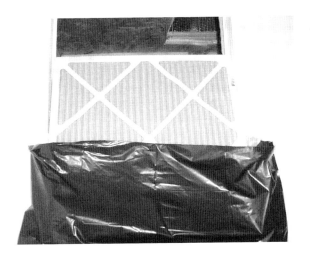

Align a properly-sized bag under the dirty filter, and slide the filter into the bag as is shown here. Some home and building staff actually carry dirty used filters throughout a home or building, dispersing mold-filled dust all over.

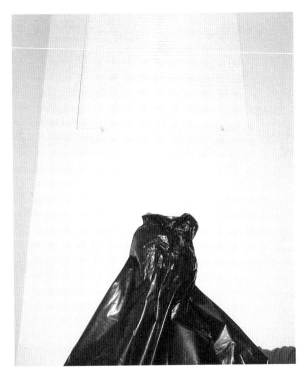

The dirty filter is slid into a very large trash bag and then closed immediately and tightly. Notice that something is missing from this bag. What do you think is floating out the top?

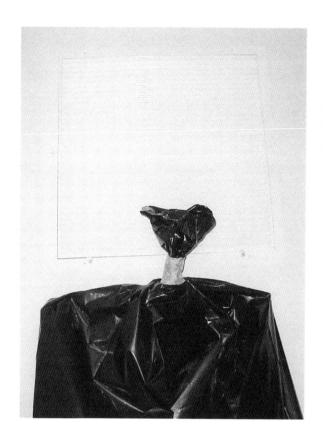

This bag is now ready to be taken out to the trash. It is sealed with strong tape. We suggest having a piece of strong tape or a very strong tie ready and available **before** you slip the filter into the bag.

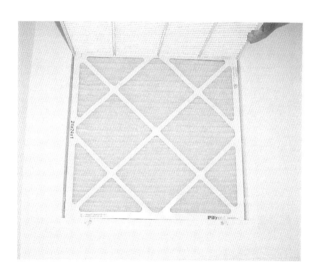

The dirty filter in now replaced with this new one. Quite a difference, huh? This white filter will now capture all sorts of mold spores, mold toxins, dust and other debris that would travel throughout a home, building or school and contaminate the AC ducts, and make people ill.

The Inexpensive N95 Mask Made Super Simple

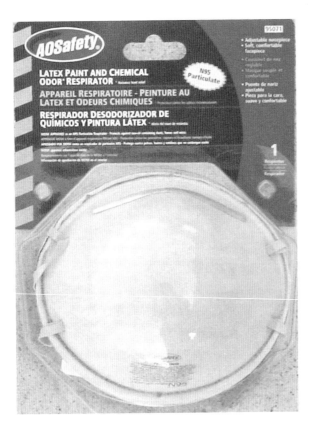 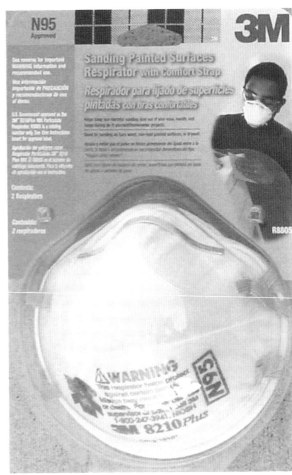

Can you see the N95 marking in two places on each package?

Note that the location of the markings are in different locations on these two sample brands. If a mask does not have the N95 designation, do not use it. Common painter's masks are worthless for mold dust protection.

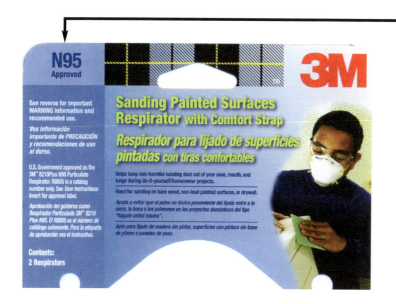

The N95 designation on the packaging.

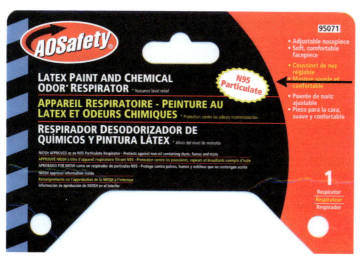

Here the designation is blown up. It is often in small print. Further, different companies use different expressions such as, "N95 Particulate," "N95 Approved" or more simply, "N95."

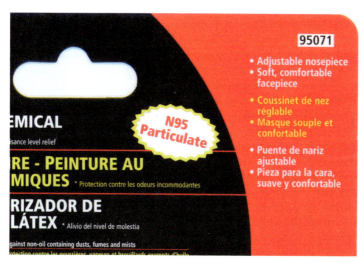

N95 Mask Markings Made Easy

When you open a mask's packaging you will probably toss it out. Later, how will you know if the mask is an N95 mask? Does the mask itself have any markings? It should.

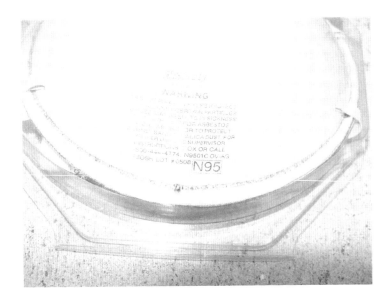

Both masks confirm the packaging, and have the printed N95 designation on the bottom or side of the mask.

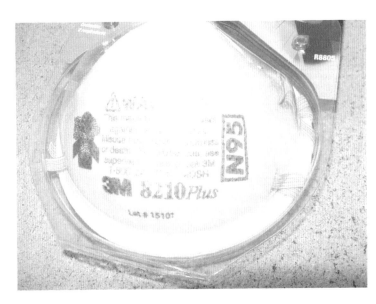

Common Junk Air Filters:
How to Make a Duct Cleaning Company Wealthy

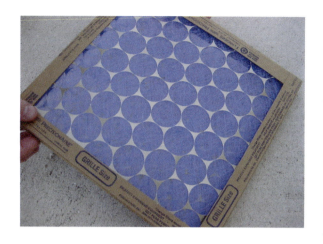

If you look in new or old homes or the ducts of different buildings, it is stunning to see these blue filters. While they look better than the equally worthless grey or black fiber filters, filters are not about looks.

How well could this filter clean air with fine mold-filled dust?

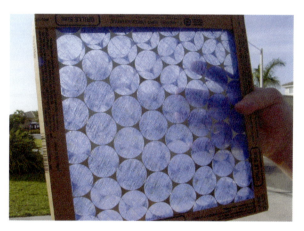

Looking at both these filters, you can see that my hand is easily visible on the underside of the filter. Meaning? If you are hoping that this pretty filter will do more than filter my hand, you will be disappointed. Replace them all with MERV 11 disposable filters, and try to have your child's school and your place of employment do the same.

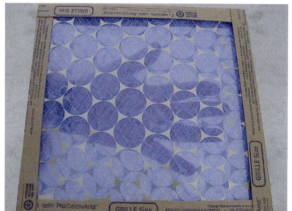

Handling Musty Moldy Books

Dr. Schaller buys about eight hundred books a year. To avoid going broke, he buys most used. Often they arrive in a group, and by the time he has opened five or six, his eyes are red and his nose is itchy.

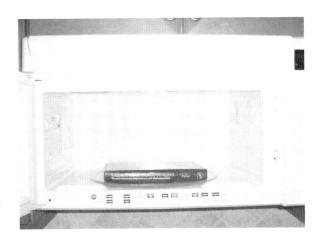

One way to kill mold on musty moldy books is to use a microwave oven. We suggest doing one book at a time for 45-60 seconds. It is possible to make the book very hot and to make the binding glue wet. If this happens, we have had good success placing the binding back to its required place, and putting some rubber bands around the book. We have yet to see any one start a fire with this approach, and we would ask you to not be our first! So do not leave any book unattended.

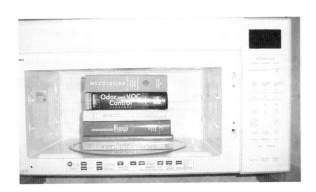

One day Dr. Schaller received a large collection of used academic books on mold. He was delighted and sat down to read them, and soon he was feeling foggy. Yes, you guessed it. The books about mold had mold – so he rushed and tossed them all into the microwave oven. Hey, but not all at once!

We cannot tell you the exact amount of time each book needs. Start with 30 seconds and add time in 30 second units until you learn how long it takes to make the book very warm, but not painfully hot to the touch. Please avoid boiling any book! A copy of Dante's Inferno might need more time then a copy of the Arctic Adventure. Finally, in an effort to diligently serve you, we called dozens of microwave manufacturers to get the "cooking time" for various books, but none returned our calls.

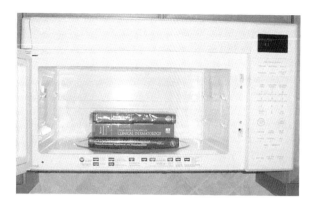

We do not suggest mixing books with plastic covers and other bindings. The plastic covered ones will get too hot, and some thick hard cover books may stay cool.

In Dr. Rosen's opinion, a microwave oven will probably kill mold spores, but it will not destroy the mold's chemical toxins. Therefore, after a musty book is "cooked" in a microwave oven, it must be fully HEPA vacuumed.

What Do Mold Labs See: A Sixty Second Introduction

Images used with permission from Edward Sobek, Ph.D,
Director of Research and Development at Clean Air Labs in Oak Ridge, TN

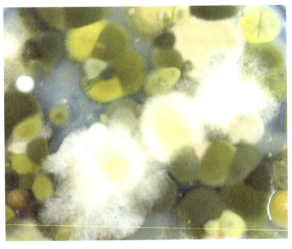

Mold from a home collected with with a machine that traps live spores.

One type of sampling device lets mold spores in the air hit a plate with growth media or mold food. The lab then grows the spores into full molds and can identify them.

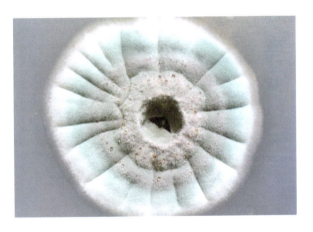

A Penicillin mold growing on a culture plate.

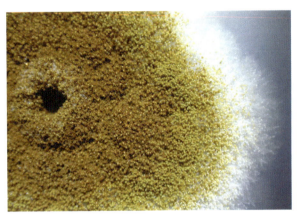

Aspergillus mold on a culture plate.

Most mold cultures do not look like what you might see in a moldy basement, attic or behind a wet wall. We suspect this is due to different "foods" and other factors. For example, drywall is not petri dish food. And the temperature used to culture mold differs from your home temperature. The most commonly found toxic indoor molds are probably toxic species of Penicillium and Aspergillus.

Basic Spore Images Used to Identify Molds

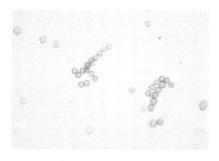

Aspergillus spores magnified only 40x

What Does A Spore Trap Show?

Most mold investigators collect "spore traps," which is a term that simply means they trap spores in the air at a set rate for a set number of minutes, so the lab can determine the number of spores per minute.

Most spore examination is done at a magnification of 600x. This image shows spores only magnified 40x. Yet, even at 600x many mold technicians have trouble distinquishing Aspergillus spores from Penicillin spores. So what is the solution?

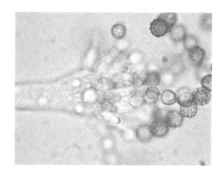

One way a lab can determine the type of mold in your home, workplace or a school is by looking at the entire structure. Here a type of Aspergillus shows a full view of many parts—the stem-like section, some branching structures and some spores. When you add all these together, the lab can determine this is Aspergillus (genus) penicillioides (species). When a lab can see the entire mold "plant," they can determine the exact species of mold, some of which are highly toxic.

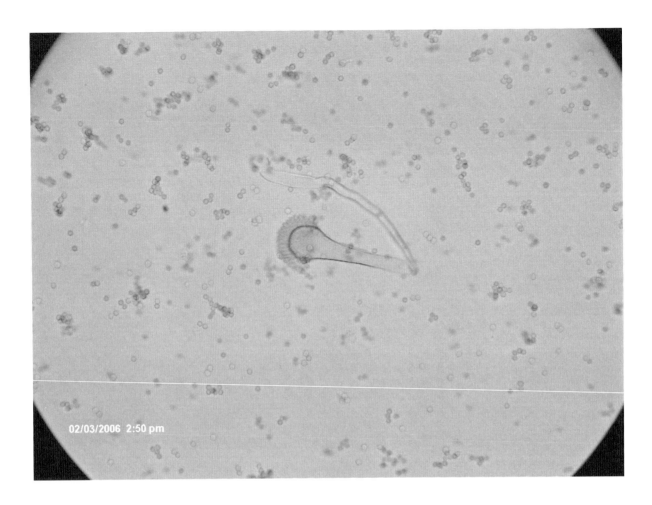

This is an image of Aspergillus fumigatus which makes mold toxins. It is often found in homes, schools and other buildings with water damage or merely excess humidity.

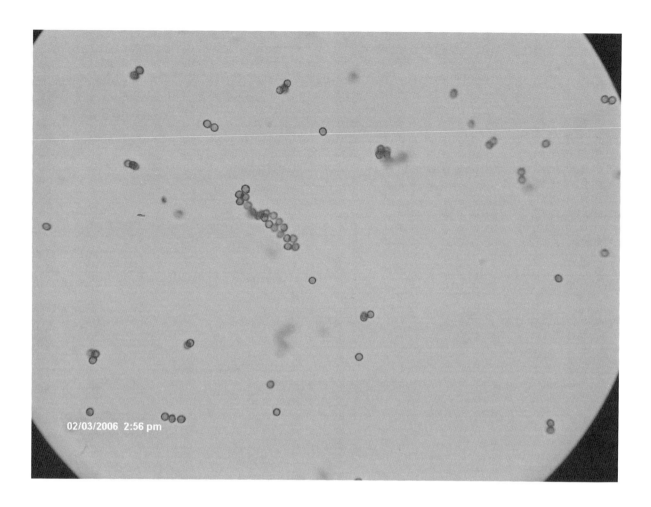

These spores are from Aspergillus niger which is a mold that makes biotoxins. Note that while the spores are the same as other Aspergillus molds (and Penicillium) spores, it has a mild black coloring. Hence the name "niger" or black.

"Black Mold" Spores

While the most common toxic molds are types of Aspergillus and Penicillium, Stachybotyrs or "black mold" is the best known in newspapers and television news reports. It does have many very potent mold toxins. Note the dark black spores.

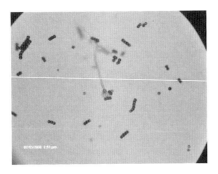

A "Cousin" of Stachybotyrs

Here is a mold related to Stachybotyrs by DNA examination. This example of Memnoniella echinata also makes biotoxins.

In this collection of spores you can see some black Stachybotyrs spores next to some light colored ones. The light colored ones could be either Aspergillus or Penicillium.

Just Because a Mold Has No Toxins Does Not Make It Healthy

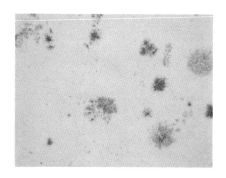

Cladosporium is very common in a moist or humid home. While it has few biotoxins, it can make patients miserable from traditional allergies. Just because some physicians are naïve about molds that make biotoxins, let's not ignore the molds that cause traditional allergies.

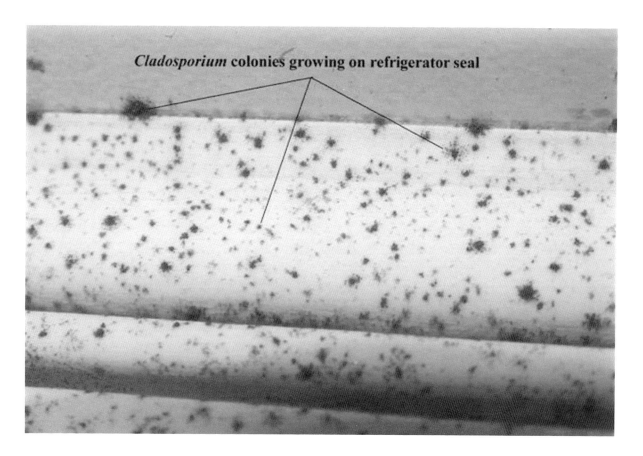

Here we see Cladosporium clearly in a refrigerator. I wonder how the owner's allergies were doing each time this was opened up? I suspect they were feeling quite uncomfortable.

Dangerous Stachybotyrs or "Black Mold"
A Glance at the Full Structure

This mold requires water and not merely high humidity to start to grow. If your lab sees images like these of "black mold" we suggest you get a well-qualified expert with at least $1M in mold insurance. The mold insurance is the only way to make sure the "expert" is qualified. The mold insurance is hard to get and only issued to qualified individuals. Certification programs are typically 2-4 day courses. Most certified individuals have no mold insurance, since they do not have the advanced training, experience and education required to qualify for mold insurance.

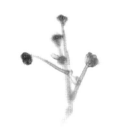

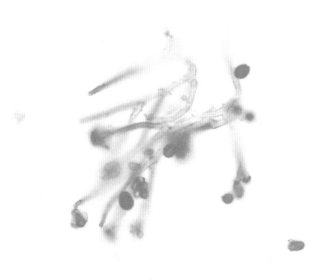

In these two images stachybotyrs' entire structure is seen.

Powerful Mold Chemicals with Weird Names

Sample toxins made by black mold:

- 3-Acetyl-deoxynivalenol
- Atranones A-G
- Cyclosporins
- Diacetoxyscirpenol
- Deoxynivalenol or Vomitoxin
- Epoxytrichothecene
- Isosatratoxins F, G & H
- Phenylspirodrimanes
- Roridins A, E
- Satratoxins F, G & H
- Stachylysin
- Trichoverrols A, B
- Verrucarins A, J
- Verrucarol (T-2-tetraol)

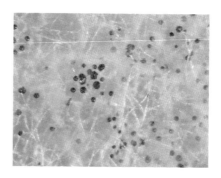

The full structure of black mold shown in a growth culture.

I wonder how many of your regular physicians have studied the effects of each of these on animals or humans.

(www.ttuhsc.edu/SOM/Microbiology/mainweb/aiaq/Glossary.html)

The Stachy or Black Mold Fetish: Missing Other Molds

Black mold is a potent toxin maker, however most building structures have mold toxins from other molds. Two important and common examples are indoor molds from the genus Aspergillus and Penicillium. The numbers of toxic mold species are vast and far outside the scope of this simple text. Most homes or structures with mold have a mix of toxic mold species, and each of these can produce a wide range of toxic substances.

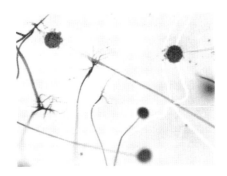

Progressive mold labs now have advanced technologies such as this polished detailed image of a Rhizopus mold (this one makes biotoxins). Another new technology is the use of DNA to look at air or dust samples to get an exact species fingerprint of the molds present in a home.

Additional Important Blood Testing Labs

Earlier in the book we mentioned some important labs which are altered by exposure to mold toxins. However, if you have insurance or can afford some additional lab testing you should consider getting these additional labs. Mold toxins alter many body chemicals, not merely MSH, VIP and Leptin.

Myelin Basic Protein

Myelin is the fat insulation on nerves. Mold and Lyme toxins can cause this insulation to be attacked by your own antibodies. This can cause you to be misdiagnosed with MS and placed on very strong medications that are missing the real cause.

If your MBP is high, it means the immune system loses control and makes antibodies that hurt the fatty nerve protection. This lab must be done at Specialty Labs and is easily sent out from LabCorp. The Specialty Lab code is 848747 with a possible diagnostic code of 340.

We have seen good results in restoring fatty nerve protection after mold remediation and mold medical care. And others improved still further with the treatment of commonly missed infections, such as Lyme, Bartonella, Ehrlichia, Babesia and Mycoplasma. Lyme, for example, can be hidden inside a wide range of human cells, which probably increases autoimmunity.

Anticardiolipin (IgA, IgG & IgM)

This lab test measures antibodies against a very specific type of cell wall fat called phospholipids. An abnormal lab result means you are attacking your own cell walls, which can cause deadly blood clots, strokes, heart attacks, and miscarriages.

Antigliadin Antibodies

Gliadin is a wheat protein that can cause intestinal irritation in some susceptible people. If mold toxins get into the body, the inflammation system can rise, causing a possible sensitivity to wheat and other common grains. Generally, after indoor mold exposure, the lab results might show the beginning of antibodies against gliadin, but the patient may not have diarrhea and severe intestinal problems yet. Any lab can do this test.

ANA with Reflex

This tests if the mold toxins have caused you to start making antibodies against your own cell nuclear material. If positive, the "reflex" means they run other tests to find out the specific types of anti-antibodies that are present. This can be done by any lab.

Homocysteine

Mold toxins sometimes consume B-Vitamins, which causes a rise in homocysteine. Most sincere physicians do not realize indoor mold can increase this dangerous amino acid. A high homocysteine triggers inflammation, injury to blood vessels, and dangerous blood clotting. This lab test is well known to physicians.

IgE

If a child or adult has asthma or allergies to a mold, the IgE level will be high. But in general, mold toxins have very little effect on IgE. If it is high, an allergist, pulmonologist, ENT, pediatrician, or family doctor could probably offer some relief, since this is a common and well-known medical problem. The toxins of mold do not cause it.

Epstein Barr Panel

We all have been exposed to this virus. So, it is assumed everyone will have results showing its presence in the blood. Some physicians feel a very high number means your immune system is not acting normally due to mold toxins or some infection hurting the immune system. Any lab can do this test. The LabCorp code is 010280 and a possible diagnostic code is 780.79.

Lab Tests Done By Quest Labs

If possible, these next two lab samples would need to be packaged in dry ice and shipped overnight to: Quest Diagnostics, 1901 Sulphur Spring Rd., Baltimore, Maryland 21227. Their phone number is 410-536-1324. Some LabCorp centers or local Quest centers will agree to send these out to Quest.

VEGF – A Critical Hormone Associated with Fatigue, Aches and Concentration

This hormone helps make new capillaries and increases blood, oxygen and sugar flow to various tissues, including the brain and muscle tissue. Some mold toxins cause abnormal levels of VEGF – either low levels or huge levels. Either extreme is bad. (The range to use in evaluating a LabCorp result is 31-115). Three common symptoms of abnormal VEGF are atypical muscle aches after exertion, fatigue and brain fog. All are likely due to the inability of VEGF to open capillaries to deliver oxygen and perhaps also glucose to the body. Abnormal levels are partially treated with high doses of Omega-3 fish oils. Two enteric coated brands that have no fish taste, and never open up in the stomach, are Fisol and a select Metagenics' product. The Quest code is 894826 and some possible diagnosis codes are 416.9, 253.2, 710.0.

Also, any youth with eccentric fatigue should be tested for an infectious agent called "Babesia" which has different varieties found throughout the United States. It is loosely related to malaria and found in different types of ticks — some smaller than a poppy-seed with painless bites. This infection is commonly missed by large mega labs with little interest in tick-born infections. We suggest testing any person having unusual fatigue with an IGeneX Babesia FISH test done along with a Babesia IgG and IgM. Some physicians think that Babesia will commonly produce urine tests showing burst red blood cells. Unfortunately, this is not always true in mild American forms. Sometimes a child can have no signs or symptoms for years. Further, adults need to be careful about justifying adolescents sleeping eleven hours a day as "growth fatigue." Adolescents do not need more than nine hours sleep each night. Also, some adults with mold or Babesia blame it on their "age." Yet, generally adults should generally not require over nine hours of sleep per day.

MMP-9

This enzyme goes up with the presence of tumors, sudden severe infections, significant inflammation and biotoxin release. Exposure to toxic mold chemicals will increase the MMP-9 level, typically over 300. It should decrease as the child or adult improves from treatment for toxin exposure. The Quest code is 821675, and one possible diagnostic code is 340.

Complement 3a or C3a

This chemical is increased during pregnancy, perhaps to increase a mother's ability to fight infection. It is a strong pro-inflammation chemical acting in at least two inflammation systems. It is seen increased in everything from unstable heart chest pain to aspirin-induced asthma. Have the samples sent to Quest Labs in Baltimore or any lab that can perform the test. The lab code is C3 4859W with a possible diagnosis of 279.8.

Future Blood Lab Research

In the previous chapters, we discuss numerous tests that might be beneficial for a diagnosis. Sample additional labs tested for adults include interleukins, inflammatory cytokines, approximately twenty hormones and autoimmune tests, C-reactive protein, and apolipoproteins. In the near future, we hope to evaluate more closely the kinin system, acetylated peptide A, PAR-2 (and related products), granzyme, perforin, and hemolysin in very select patients who are not improving.

Binders, Binders and More Mold Toxin Binders

The most popular mold toxin binder is a prescription medication called, "cholestyramine." It binds mold toxins in the intestinal track and prevents them from being absorbed. Currently, it is available by prescription in packets or a small container dispensed with a scoop. We routinely have it compounded, so that the sugar and artificial coloring is removed. It can be made with xylitol, which is a slow-release healthy sugar, and a wide range of minerals like magnesium and zinc to prevent constipation. In rare cases, a 1/4 teaspoon of magnesium citrate (or higher) will almost always relieve constipation, but we prefer to use poorly absorbed healthy minerals first.

Children usually take one dose of cholestyramine per day, and adolescents take two doses a day. Adults should take four doses a day. This medication should not be taken with food or medications, because it will just bind them. We usually like patients to take important medications an hour before a dose. It is possible to take a dose every hour. Some adults take packets to work and take them every hour after lunch. Some patients prefer to take their cholestyramine in capsules. We prescribe 400 mg, 600 mg and 800 mg capsules with pure cholestyramine resin. Therefore, a "dose" will mean taking about 6-10 capsules per dose, depending on the capsule size.

Also, these capsules are usually not covered by insurance and are at least $250.00 per month.

If a patient has significant nausea and indigestion with cholestyramine there are many treatment options. Some people use over-the-counter or prescription antacid medications which might be effective for mold toxin stomach erosion or irritation. Cholestyramine itself can annoy some stomachs and **we have had success starting with the lowest amount tolerable**. Some patients with nausea or indigestion are helped by the addition of prescription Carafate which coats the stomach and is an old ulcer medication.

College Pharmacy in Colorado has made a special enterically-coated cholestyramine capsule which dissolves as soon as it exits the stomach. We have not been able to research this product yet.

Other mold toxin binders are also used by some clinicians and mold remediators. Welchol comes in prescription tablets which are covered by most insurance plans, but it is weaker than cholestyramine. Activated pharmaceutical charcoal capsules are felt to bind some mold toxins, but miss others. Chitosan is rumored to be a cheap over-the-counter mold toxin binder, but Dr. Ritchie Shoemaker, a prolific biotoxin researcher working near a chitosan production plant, has not found it to be successful. He feels that virtually any stomach acid may limit its ability to bind mold toxins. Many other binders are used in alternative medicine, in animal feeds and in grain processing. Discussing each is outside our scope.

Dr. Schaller is doing research looking at many of these substances used to bind mold toxins. Perhaps some day he will be able to use DNA home samples to target both the mold species and the mold toxin, and then to target a special binder to fit each person's specific exposure.

New Home and Building Denaturing Agents

Dr. Schaller is researching a wide range of natural and synthetic chemicals for safe ways to denature or destroy mold biotoxins. These biotoxins must be removed or destroyed in moldy homes or other buildings. This research includes new safe products that will only act when mold is present. This research will be available at www.usmoldphysician.com when it is completed.

Increasing the Body's Ability to Remove Biotoxins

About 25% of the population is inefficient at removing mold toxins "naturally." Using research on genetic mutations, Dr. Schaller is looking at ways to increase the body's ability to overcome its limited ability to remove biotoxins. Some think this is as simple as taking glutathione or a liver detox product. While these are important products for overall health, Dr. Schaller is looking into targeting exact toxic mold species or their mycotoxins from a contaminated building by DNA identification, and then adding very high doses of specific nutritional substances. The goal is to promote the exact liver reaction that will remove specific mold toxins found in a home or other structure. This information will be published on Dr. Schaller's web sites or on Amazon.com as it is completed.

Diseases and the Clothing They Wear

Transplant physicians have used cell surface proteins or cell markers to match organ transplants between individuals for decades. Scientists also discovered that these same cell markers can be found in certain diseases. If you think of cell markings like "clothing" then if a person had a certain pattern, they were at higher risk to develop a certain disease. Using our clothing analogy, a person wearing black leather is rarely a kindergarten teacher. The clothes "make" or give us insight into the man, and the cell's outer markers or "clothing" give us insight into the cell.

Dr. Shoemaker used this type of testing in thousands of patients and found very clear patterns regarding mold toxin removal. He found that about twenty-five percent of the U.S. population does not properly remove mold toxins. If they were exposed to low levels of mold toxins, toxins are collected in their bodies and over time can make these individuals more and more ill.

We found the same patterns in our research. The cell marker results fit exactly with other abnormal lab results and the severity of mold illness. This is very progressive medicine, and slowly more and more physicians are learning how to do this type of analysis.

In the book **Mold Warriors: Fighting American's Hidden Health Threat**, there are some tools for interpreting the HLA patterns. Additionally, depending on availability, either Dr. Schaller or Dr. Shoemaker, or both can evaluate your HLA results and return to you an HLA results chart with your pattern clearly circled.

The cost for this service is $35.00 which will be used to fund further health care publications by the Shoemaker and Schaller team.

Simply send your results to Dr. Schaller. His mailing address can be found on his primary web site at www.personalconsult.com.

Enclose a check for $35 made out to: James Schaller, M.D.

Or go to the www.personalconsult.com home page and pay $35.00 by credit card where it reads, "Make a payment." Allow two weeks for processing.

This special test to determine your ability to remove biotoxins is only done by a top national lab, LabCorp. The test name and LabCorp code is: HLA DRB, DBQ Disease Evaluation 012542. Some physicians use the following diagnostic codes: 279.10, 377.34, 279.8.

Other Sample Mold Books by Drs. Rosen and Schaller

When Traditional Medicine Fails ...

Available at your local bookstore, or online at Amazon.com

Revised 2nd Edition

Parents are calling this book "Miraculous" because it works...when all else has failed.

When Traditional Medicine Fails...

Your Guide to

MOLD TOXINS

- What they are.
- Who they hurt.
- And what <u>you</u> can do to reclaim your child's health, learning and behavior.

Gary Rosen, Ph.D., C.I.E.
James Schaller, M.D., C.M.R.

Includes Home Detox Program

Dr. Schaller is the co-author of this 600 page medical text on mold illness.

It is available from Amazon.com

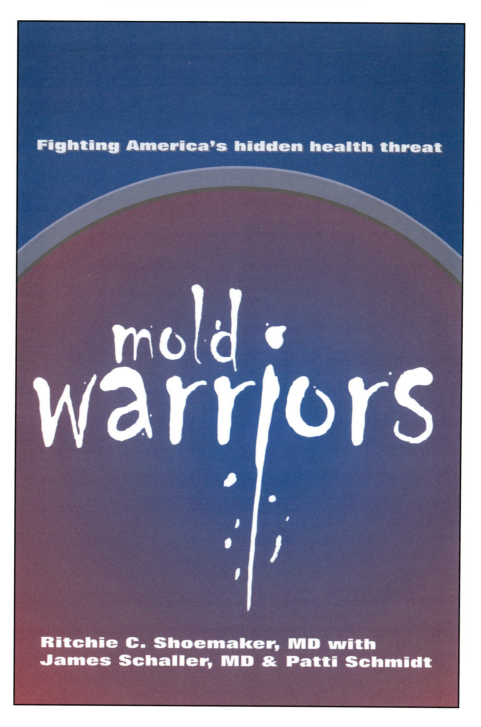

The medical ideas, health thoughts, building health comments, products and any claims made about specific illnesses, diseases, and causes of health problems in this book, have not been evaluated by the FDA, the USDA, OSHA, CDC, NIH, NIMH or the AMA. Never assume any United States medical body or society, or the majority of American physicians endorse any comment in this book. No comments in this book are approved by any government agency or medical body or society. No comments in this book are meant to diagnose, treat, cure or prevent disease. The information provided in this book is for informational purposes only and is not intended as a substitute for the advice from your physician or other health care professional. This book is not intended to replace or adjust any information contained on or in any product label or packaging. You should not use the information in this book for the diagnosis or treatment of any health problem or as an endorsement of any prescription medication or other treatment. You should consult with a health care professional before deciding on any diagnosis, or initiating any treatment plan of any kind. Please do not start any diet, exercise or supplementation program, or take any type of nutrient, herb, or medication without clear consultation with your licensed health care provider. If you have or suspect you might have a health problem, please do not use this book to replace a prompt consultation with your health care provider(s).